Workbook for

Surgical Technology:
Principles and Practice

Workbook for

Surgical Technology: Principles and Practice

Eighth Edition

Prepared by

Elizabeth Ness, CST, BA
Program Coordinator
Surgical Technology
Macomb Community College
Clinton Township, Michigan

ELSEVIER

Elsevier
3251 Riverport Lane
St. Louis, Missouri 63043

WORKBOOK FOR SURGICAL TECHNOLOGY, EIGHTH EDITION   ISBN: 9780323935333

Notice

Practitioners and researchers must always rely on their own experience and knowledge in evaluating
and using any information, methods, compounds or experiments described herein. Because of rapid
advances in the medical sciences, in particular, independent verification of diagnoses and drug dosages
should be made. To the fullest extent of the law, no responsibility is assumed by Elsevier, authors, editors
or contributors for any injury and/or damage to persons or property as a matter of products liability,
negligence or otherwise, or from any use or operation of any methods, products, instructions, or ideas
contained in the material herein.

Previous editions copyrighted 2018, 2015, 2012, 2009, 2005, 2002, and 1999

International Standard Book Number: 9780323935333

Senior Content Strategist: Nancy O'Brien
Content Development Specialist: Elizabeth McCormac
Publishing Services Manager: Shereen Jameel
Project Manager: Aparna Venkatachalam

Printed in India

Last digit is the print number: 9   8   7   6   5   4   3   2

Working together
to grow libraries in
developing countries

www.elsevier.com • www.bookaid.org

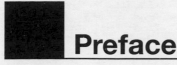

Preface

This new edition of the Workbook has been written to solidify a student's awareness of his or her grasp of the topics presented in *Surgical Technology: Principles and Practice*, eighth edition. The questions have been specifically designed to challenge students' strategic thinking skills and to get them to think creatively about scenarios that are commonplace in the modern operating room. The following exercises have been used to meet these goals:

- **Key Terms**. The most important key terms are presented to enhance clarification. Students are asked to differentiate between two terms that are commonly confused and whose precise definitions are key to understanding important concepts.
- **Short Answer** questions apply knowledge learned from the text to a variety of situations.

- **Matching:** These exercises allow students to define and categorize words within a specific area of surgical technology practice. This in turn enhances memorization of each term's meaning and significance.
- **Multiple choice** questions provide a way to differentiate and define information.
- **Labeling** exercises reinforce important anatomy concepts that a surgical technologist should be familiar with.
- **Case Studies** have been carefully written to improve students' critical thinking skills and challenge them to look at clinical situations from various points of view. The case studies also provide a basis for group discussion and knowledge sharing.
- **Skills Checklists** provide clear guidelines on how skills should be performed and help students self-evaluate the performance of core functions by practicing skills.

Contents

Workbook for

Surgical Technology: Principles and Practice

1 Surgical Technology: The Profession and the Professional

Student's Name _____

KEY TERMS

Write the definition for each term.

1. ABHES: _____

2. ACS: _____

3. Allied health profession: _____

4. AHA: _____

5. AMA: _____

6. ANSI: _____

7. ARC/STSA: _____

8. ASA: _____

9. AST: _____

10. Certification: _____

11. Continuing education: _____

12. CST: _____

13. CST-CFA: _____

14. Nonsterile team members: _____

15. ORT: _____

16. Professional characteristics: _____

17. Proprietary school: _____

18. Scrub: _____

19. Sterile personnel: _____

20. Surgical conscience: _____

21. STSR: _____

COMPUTER ASSIGNMENT

Research what the abbreviations for following organizations stand for and what each of them is responsible for.

1. AORN: _____

_____

2. ARC/STSA: _____

_____

3. CAAHEP: _____

_____

4. NBSTSA: _____

_____

SHORT ANSWERS

Provide a short answer for each question or statement.

1. What is an ethical dilemma?

_____

_____

2. What are the educational options for students who want to be surgical technologists?

_____

_____

3. Why is it important for a practicing surgical technologist to engage in continued education?

_____

_____

4. Name areas of potential employment for a graduate surgical technologist.

_____

_____

5. List career opportunities for surgical technologists.

_____

_____

6. Surgical conscience is a specific set of professional attributes that are associated with surgery; define:

Accountability _____

_____

Confidentiality _____

_____

7. List professional ethics for health care workers.

_____

_____

_____

8. What are the characteristics of a professional?

_____

_____

9. What types of support and services are provided by AST?

_____

_____

_____

MATCHING

Match the following individuals with a description of their roles. Individuals may have multiple roles, and each question may have more than one answer.

_____ 1. Maintain retraction of tissue

_____ 2. Scrub, gown, and glove self and team members

_____ 3. Communicate effectively with surgeon to prevent errors

_____ 4. Nonsterile team member who acts as an advocate for the patient and provides assistance to the sterile surgical team

_____ 5. Performs surgical maneuvers such as cutting tissue, maintaining hemostasis, and suturing under the direction of the primary surgeon

_____ 6. Specialist in the preparation, handling, and use of instruments

_____ 7. Prepares medications and solutions for use in the surgical wound

_____ 8. Teaches new employees and surgical technology students in surgery

_____ 9. Pursues an advanced degree in hospital administration and management

_____ 10. Trained in the processes of disinfection, inspection, assembly, and sterilization of instrument trays

_____ 11. Maintains a "dry" surgical site by operating suction devices and appropriate use of surgical sponge

_____ 12. Ensures patient chart, including results of diagnostic procedures, permits, and preoperative checklist, accompany the patient in surgery

_____ 13. Prepares instruments and supplies on the sterile field

_____ 14. Nonsterile person who completes documentation, performs skin prep, urinary catheterization, and assists in positioning the patient on the operating table

_____ 15. Assists in hemostatis by clamping blood vessels and securing them with suture

_____ 16. Assists surgeon in specific, well-defined tasks as needed during a procedure

a. Surgical technologist

b. Circulator

c. CST-CFA First Assistant

d. Preceptor

e. Second assistant

f. Leadership and management

MULTIPLE CHOICE

1. The surgical technologist working in a hospital or other facility that provides 24-hour care is usually required to:
   a. Work a double shift
   b. Work a 24 hour shift
   c. Work over time
   d. Be on "call"

2. All of the following are areas for graduate surgical technologists to work except:
   a. Hospitals
   b. Ambulatory surgery center
   c. RN OR educator
   d. Specialty practice

3. Reliability, trustworthiness, responsibility and honesty are all examples of which of the following?
   a. Self-regulation
   b. Integrity
   c. Tactfulness
   d. Respect for rules, regulations, and laws

4. Which of the following is one of the best known ethical standards in medicine?
   a. Ethical dilemma
   b. Empathy
   c. Practice equal rights
   d. Do no harm

5. Which of the following refers to a professional's accountability by admitting any mistakes immediately to prevent harm to the patient.
   a. Surgical conscience
   b. Commitment
   c. Tact and discression
   d. Sclf-regulation

CASE STUDIES

1. *Read the following case study and answer the questions based on your knowledge of the scope of practice for a surgical technologist:*

   You are a new student in the operating room. Halfway through the procedure you think you notice a tear in the sleeve of your gown. It is a very small tear and not very visible, and you are not sure what to do because you will be embarrassed and do not want to get in trouble. You do not think anyone will notice the tear.

   a. What should you do in this situation?

   b. Will you get in trouble?

2 Communication and Teamwork

Student's Name _____

KEY TERMS

1. Assertiveness: _____

2. Body language: _____

3. Consensus: _____

4. Facilitator: _____

5. Feedback: _____

6. Gossip: _____

7. Groupthink: _____

8. Message: _____

9. Norms: _____

10. Receiver: _____

11. Rumor: _____

12. Sender: _____

13. Therapeutic touch: _____

14. Win-lose solution: _____

15. Win-win solution: _____

SHORT ANSWERS

Provide a short answer for each question or statement.

1. What are the elements of positive listening skills?

_____

_____

2. What environmental barriers to good communication are common in the operating room?

_____

_____

3. When is communication considered successful?

_____

_____

MATCHING

Match each term with the correct definition regarding successful communication. Some terms may be used more than once.

_____ 1. Expressing one's own needs and rights while respecting the needs and rights of others.

_____ 2. Polite concise language without sany rudeness directed respectfully towards the other person.

_____ 3. Reporting a problem or situation to appropriate personnel, not to someone who does not have any control of the situation.

_____ 4. The message delivered is concise and to the point.

_____ 5. Taking consideration the person, time and place when communicating a need in reporting an event or situation.

_____ 6. Shifting gaze on the other person from one eye to the other.

_____ 7. A message that carries no emotion.

_____ 8. The message is delivered in simple, straight forward language that is understood by those receiving it.

a. Conciseness

b. Assertiveness

c. Neutrality

d. Clarity

e. Right person, right time, right place

f. Civility

g. Follow chain of command

h. Maintain eye contact

MATCHING

Choose from the terms of methods of communication failure listed and match them with their most correct description. You may use an answer more than once.

_____ 1. Personal views may not coincide with others, making assumptions of what is seen heard and understood based on our views.

_____ 2. How we perceive a problem, situation, or action sometimes depends on our social and cultural background as much as our knowledge.

_____ 3. A preexisting opinion about people based on affiliations, culture, economic status and disease.

_____ 4. How we feel at the time of communication, can effect the ability to send and receive messages.

_____ 5. Receiver does not have sufficient knowledge to understand exactly what the sender is trying to communicate.

_____ 6. Hearing is a particular problem in the operating room, background noises and muffled speech are all examples of:

_____ 7. To be successful in sending and receiving information, a person must want to communicate.

_____ 8. Skill and knowledge to communicate and integrate well with people from diverse backgrounds.

a. Cultural competence

b. Emotions

c. Environmental barriers

d. Lack of a desire to communicate

e. Perception of the situation

f. Bias

g. Lack of understanding

h. Social and cultural influences

8

MULTIPLE CHOICE

Choose the most correct answer to complete the question or statement.

1. Communication should take place with the:
   a. Right person, time, and place
   b. Right time, person, and situation
   c. Right situation, person, and place
   d. Right person, place, and things

2. Who is the "right person" to communicate a problem within the workplace?
   a. Top management in all situations so that you are sure the message reaches the most authoritative person
   b. Someone who seems to have the right answers most of the time
   c. One who can sympathize with the problem
   d. One who has the authority to help solve the problem

3. _____ maintains appropriate social boundaries when speaking to patients in the health care environment.
   a. A professional
   b. A department manager
   c. An instructor
   d. Someone who is mature in age

4. The professional understands that most patients _____.
   a. Are naturally concerned and worried
   b. Do not understand the surgery or its risks
   c. Have a high respect for health care workers
   d. Are well informed about the surgery, since they must sign the surgical consent

5. The operating room requires its personnel to work at a high level of mental, physical, and emotional strength. Because of this environment, the work is:
   a. Necessary
   b. Good
   c. Stressful
   d. Rehearsed

6. When working with people with problem behaviors, one must remember to focus on the behavior and not the _____.
   a. Person
   b. Attitude
   c. Team
   d. Task

7. A _____ is a group of people who come together to reach a common goal or set of goals.
   a. Gang
   b. Team
   c. Professional
   d. None of the above

8. Most role confusion is a result of poor:
   a. Teamwork
   b. Groupthink
   c. Attitude
   d. Communication

9. The goal of conflict resolution is to attempt to find a solution that is acceptable to all parties; this is called a _____-_____ solution.
   a. Win lose
   b. Win win
   c. Conflict resolution
   d. Open minded

10. In the role of _____, the surgical technologist tutors the student and shares the duties of a scrubbed technologist.
    a. Team leader
    b. Preceptor
    c. Manager
    d. Instructor

CASE STUDIES

1. *Read the following scenario and then answer the questions that follow:*

You are in the operating room and scrubbed in for an exploratory laparotomy. The anesthesiologist and your circulator are chatting about a movie they both recently saw. The surgeon remains focused on the field. At this point there is increased hemorrhage and the surgery becomes more intense. You interrupt the circulator in her conversation to alert her to the sudden hemorrhage, and ask for more sponges.

After the patient has been taken to the postanesthesia care unit (PACU) and is stable, your circulator comes to you and states that you made her look "stupid" in front of the surgeon and the anesthesiologist.

a. Is the circulator's evaluation of the situation valid?

b. How do you respond to her?

c. What is the real issue here, and does it matter who is right?

3 Medicolegal Aspects of Surgical Technology

Student's Name _____

KEY TERMS

Write the definition for each term.

1. Abandonment: _____

2. Accountability: _____

3. Administrative law: _____

4. Advance directive: _____

5. Adverse event: _____

6. Certification: _____

7. Damages: _____

8. Defamation: _____

9. Delegation: _____

10. Evidenced-based practice: _____

11. Hospital policy: _____

12. Incident report: _____

13. Informed consent: _____

14. Lateral abuse: _____

15. Laws: _____

16. Libel: _____

17. Licensure: _____

18. Malpractice: _____

19. Medical power of attorney: _____

20. Negligence: _____

21. Perjury: _____

22. Practice acts: _____

23. Registration: _____

11

24. Regulations: _____

25. Retained foreign object: _____

26. Sentinel event: _____

27. Sexual harassment: _____

28. Slander: _____

29. Standard of conduct: _____

30. Statutes: _____

31. Subpoena: _____

32. TIMEOUT: _____

33. Tort: _____

34. Unretrieved device fragment: _____

35. Vertical abuse: _____

SHORT ANSWERS

Provide a short answer for each question or statement.

1. Describe a sentinel event and what categorizes something as a sentinel event.

   _____

   _____

2. What are the requirements for the delegation of a task?

   _____

   _____

3. What is accountability, and how does it apply to the surgical technologist's role in the health care facility?

   _____

   _____

4. What does the Latin phrase *respondeat superior* mean?

   _____

   _____

5. Who is responsible when a delegated task results in patient harm or injury?

   _____

   _____

6. In legal terms, what does it mean for a person to "do no harm"? Contrast that with what it means to the operating room team to "do no harm." Are they the same?

_____

_____

7. Can an approved hospital policy contradict the law of the state?

_____

_____

8. What is negligence?

_____

_____

9. What are the four elements of negligence that must be proven in a lawsuit?

_____

_____

10. Why is documentation so important? Explain the medical consequences of poor documentation.

_____

_____

11. How does lateral abuse affect the work environment?

_____

_____

12. How can the receiver of verbal abuse approach the abuser?

_____

_____

13. How do you deal with problem behaviors in the operating room?

_____

_____

14. What is sexual harassment, and how does one deal with it in the operating room?

_____

_____

15. Bullying is the most common abusive behavior in health care. It is defined by The Joint Commission as:

_____

_____

_____

16. List The Joint Commission five categories of work place violence.

1. _____

2. _____

3. _____

4. _____

5. _____

MATCHING

Choose from the terms listed and match them with their most correct description. You may use the same answer more than once.

_____ 1. Legal principles or rules established through legal precedents

_____ 2. Create standards that meet or exceed Joint Commission requirements.

_____ 3. State laws.

_____ 4. Violation may result in disciplinary action by the facility.

_____ 5. Regulations passed by agencies and departments of the government such as the FDA and OSHA.

_____ 6. Practice acts.

_____ 7. Created by specialists within the organization in consultation with The Joint Commission to create best practices.

_____ 8. State and federal laws that make specific behaviors illegal.

_____ 9. Laws that protect the right of individuals.

_____ 10. Rules established by the Environmental Protection Agency (EPA) for the handling of medical waste.

_____ 11. Branch of law that applies previous legal decisions to a case currently being judged.

_____ 12. Types of government law responsible for many agencies that administer laws having to do with health care including Health Insurance Portability and Accountability Act (HIPPA) and Medicare insurance.

a. Hospital policy

b. Statutes

c. Administrative law

d. Legal doctrines

e. Common law

f. Criminal law

g. Federal law

h. Civil law

MULTIPLE CHOICE

Choose the correct answer for the question or statement.

1. You are scrubbed on a case in which the surgeons are discussing the patient's personal affairs that have no bearing on the surgical procedure or medical condition. These comments make you feel uncomfortable; you would consider this:
   a. Not your concern
   b. Lateral abuse
   c. Sexual harassment
   d. Slander

2. Tammy is a program director who frequently talks about her supervisor. Tammy informs the class that her supervisor is uneducated and does not know the standards and guidelines. These comments are:
   a. Defamation
   b. Negligent
   c. Assault
   d. Slander

3. _____ means deliberate efforts to erode the reputation of another person.
   a. Defamation
   b. Assault
   c. Battery
   d. Slander

4. _____ is the threat or attempt to harm another person.
   a. Battery
   b. False imprisonment
   c. Assault
   d. Slander

5. _____ involves contact with intent to injure and applies even if no injury occurred.
   a. Battery
   b. False imprisonment
   c. Assault
   d. Slander

6. Restraints become a method of managing a group of patients all in one place, possibly against their will. This type of case might be considered as:
   a. Battery
   b. False imprisonment
   c. Assault
   d. Slander

7. HIPAA protects a patient's _____ and other health information through its privacy rule.
   a. Medical records
   b. Opinions
   c. Legal record including past convictions
   d. Constitutional rights

8. _____ represent a permanent legal record of the patient's interaction with health care providers and services.
   a. Laboratory results
   b. Surgical consent
   c. Documentation
   d. Forms

9. The _____ is the process in which the attending practitioner explains the risks, benefits, and alternatives of the surgery to the patient.
   a. Health literacy
   b. Signed consent
   c. Informed consent
   d. Discharge criteria

10. The surgical consent is signed by the _____.
    a. Nurse and anesthesiologist
    b. Surgeon and surgical technologist
    c. Patient, surgeon, and witness
    d. Patient, PCA, and surgeon

11. If a patient is mentally incompetent or incapacitated, who may sign the informed consent on behalf of the patient?
    a. A responsible guardian
    b. An agency representative
    c. A court representative
    d. All of the above

12. Which of the following legal doctrines represents *Res ipsa loquitor*?
    a. "Let the master respond"
    b. "The thing speaks for itself"
    c. "First do no harm"
    d. Doctrine of foreseeability

13. In an effort to prevent harm to the patient, the health professional should be able to predict specific risks associated with their duties that could injure the patient. Which of the following legal doctrines is this?
    a. *Primum non nocere*
    b. *Res ipsa loquitor*
    c. *Respondeat superior*
    d. Doctrine of forseeability

14. What is the most frequent cause of injury in the operating room?
    a. Burns
    b. Falls
    c. Incorrect patient positioning
    d. Wrong site surgery

15. While transporting a patient to the OR, the circulator realized she left the patient's oxygen tank in pre-op holding. She leaves the patient on the gurney in the hallway outside the door to the OR while she runs to get the O_2 tank; meanwhile the patient needed to use the restroom and tried to get off the gurney and fell on the floor. Which of the following is the circulator charged with?
    a. Assault
    b. Battery
    c. Abandonment
    d. Slander

16. Verbal abuse is a significant problem in the _____.
    a. Professional environment
    b. Operating room
    c. Family and work
    d. Work environment

17. What is verbal abuse?
    a. Vulgar remarks
    b. Violent public criticism demeaning another person
    c. Loud and abrasive comments or demands
    d. All of the ablve

18. Verbal abuse sometimes is built into the operating room _____.
    a. Culture
    b. Environment
    c. Management
    d. Surgeons

19. Most people are reluctant to report abuse in the workplace for fear of:
    a. Retaliation
    b. Losing their job
    c. More abuse
    d. Embarassment

20. _____ abuse takes place among staff members of equal rank and position.
    a. Lateral
    b. Verbal
    c. Vertical
    d. Physical

21. Sexual harassment is an extreme abuse of power in which a person engages in the following types of behavior:
    a. Expects sexual favors in exchange for personal or professional gain
    b. Directs sexually explicit comments toward another
    c. Directs vulgar of sexual innuendoes at another
    d. All of the above

22. Victims of sexual harassment should confront the perpetrator when sexual harassment occurs and afterward submit:
    a. A written report
    b. An oral report
    c. Nothing
    d. A warning to everyone in the department

23. Which of the following intentional torts would involve publicly discussing or depicting patients outside the health care environment?
    a. Defamation
    b. Assault
    c. Libel
    d. Invasion of privacy

24. Which of the following is a deliberate effort to erode the reputation of another person in a written form?
    a. Incident form
    b. Slander
    c. Libel
    d. Hospital policy

25. When handling the surgical specimen careful handling and documentation are essential; which of the following could happen if an error occured with improper labeling or loss of specimen?
    a. Disastrous consequences for the patient
    b. Delay in treatment
    c. Misdiagnosis
    d. All of the above

CASE STUDIES

1. *Read the following case study and answer the questions based on your knowledge of unintentional torts or civil wrongs.*

   You have just been served with legal documents that suggest that you were scrubbed in on a procedure in which your patient was burned. You are charged with negligence. For what reasons could you be charged with negligence in this situation?

2. You are a student who is about to graduate and is offered a job at your extern site. The surgeon you are working with is making sexual comments that make you uncomfortable.

   a. What should you do?

   b. Why is documentation so important in issues involving sexual harassment?

   c. Is this sexual harassment?

   d. How do you know it is sexual harassment/

3. *Read the following case study and answer the questions based on your knowledge of the scope and practice for a surgical technologist:*

You are a surgical technologist who has been hired as a new graduate in the local surgery center. You have worked there for about a month, and a seasoned certified surgical technologist is still acting as your preceptor. You have been assigned to work with Dr. Smith, who will be performing an open inguinal hernia procedure. You have never worked with this surgeon before. Once the procedure begins, the surgeon asks you to administer the local anesthetic. You know that as a surgical technologist, you are not allowed to administer medications.

a. Are you performing tasks delegated by the surgeon?

b. Is administration of a local anesthetic within your scope of practice?

c. Can you perform this task if the surgeon states that he will take the responsibility?

d. What should you do in this situation?

4 Health Care Facility Structure and Environment

Student's Name _____

KEY TERMS

Write the definition for each term.

1. Accreditation (of a health care facility): _____

2. Administration: _____

3. AHRQ: _____

4. AIA: _____

5. APIC: _____

6. Back table: _____

7. Biomedical engineering technician: _____

8. Case cart system: _____

9. Central core: _____

10. Chain of command: _____

11. Decontamination area: _____

12. Efficiency: _____

13. EPA: _____

14. Integrated operating room: _____

15. Job description: _____

16. Job title: _____

17. OSHA: _____

18. Personnel policy: _____

19. Postanesthesia care unit (PACU): _____

20. Risk management: _____

21. Semirestricted area: _____

22. The Joint Commission: _____

23. Traffic patterns: _____

19

24. Transitional area: _____

25. Unrestricted area: _____

SHORT ANSWERS

Provide a short answer for each question or statement.

1. The surgical department is structured and engineered with three objectives in mind. List the three objectives.

   a. _____

   b. _____

   c. _____

2. Traffic patterns in the operating room are restricted. Describe the typical traffic pattern for an operating room, and explain why the movement is restricted.

   _____

   _____

3. Name two basic principles of infection control used in the physical design of the operating room.

   _____

   _____

   _____

4. List departments that support the operating room.

   _____

   _____

   _____

   _____

5. Who is the operating room educator, and what are the job duties of this person in the operating room?

   _____

   _____

6. Describe the chain of command and give an example of why the chain of command is important for communicating within the department.

   _____

   _____

7. Design an operating room suite to include all ancillary areas and locations the following areas may be located. Include the following areas:
   Surgical waiting area, urgical offices, locker room, employee lounge, pre-op patient care holding area, scrub sinks, sterile instrument storage room, central core, equipment storage, decontamination, clean processing area, anesthesia department, and PACU

Match each term with the correct definition. Some terms may be used more than once.

_____ 1. Answers phone, relays messages within the surgical department. During emergency, assists management with rescheduling procedures and notifying all personnel of changes.

_____ 2. The patients primary physician in the operating room.

_____ 3. Provides direct patient care of daily living, including assisting with mobility, dressing, eating and toileting.

_____ 4. Specialist in performing procedures and tests measuring brain activity.

_____ 5. Prepares the sterile field, assists surgeon with draping, passing instruments, and accountability for all items in the sterile field used in surgery.

_____ 6. Performs diagnostic imaging procedures of patients, including x-ray, CT, and MRI.

_____ 7. Maintain meticulous assessment, monitoring, and adjustments of the patient's physiological status during surgery.

_____ 8. Performs circulating duties.

_____ 9. Provides extracorporeal (outside the body) oxygenation of the blood during cardiac bypass procedures.

_____ 10. Disinfection, decontamination, inspection, assembly, and sterilization of instruments and supplies.

_____ 11. Provides exposure, hemostasis, suturing, suctioning, and other tasks assigned by the surgeon.

a. Certified Surgical Technologist (CST)

b. Perfusionist

c. Anesthesia Provider

d. Perioperative Registered Nurse

e. Unit Clerk

f. Certified Surgical Technologist - Certified Surgical First Assistant (CST-CFA)

g. Surgeon

h. Patient Care Technician

i. Central Processing Technician

j. Radiology Technician

k. Electroencephalogram (EEG) Technician

MATCHING

Choose from the terms listed and match them with their most correct description. You may use the same answer more than once.

_____ 1. Adjustable for height, degree of tilt in all directions used for positioning the patient.

_____ 2. Large, stainless steel table on which all instruments and supplies except those in immediate use are placed.

_____ 3. Small tables used for skin prep kits, power equipment, and extra sterile supplies that may be too heavy or bulky to place or open on to the back table.

_____ 4. Smaller table with one open end that can be raised and lowered.

_____ 5. The surface is covered with a firm removable pad.

_____ 6. Holds wrapped basin sets.

_____ 7. Designated for soiled surgical sponges.

_____ 8. Is covered with a sterile drape and used for instruments and supplies that are needed immediately during surgery.

_____ 9. Before surgery a sterile pack is opened on this table containing table covers, drapes, towels and gowns.

_____ 10. Is designed to support the lip of the basin.

a. Back table

b. Mayo stand

c. Ring stand

d. Kick bucket

e. Prep tables

f. Operating room table

MULTIPLE CHOICE

Choose the most correct answer to complete the question or statement.

1. _____ is the economic use of time and energy to save unnecessary work, material resources, and time.
   a. Efficiency
   b. Engineering
   c. Environment
   d. Operations

2. _____ are physical routes for people and equipment in the health care facility, which are designed to prevent the transmission of disease.
   a. Airflow
   b. Traffic patterns
   c. Clean area
   d. Certain areas

3. The department is separated into three distinct areas:
   a. Restricted, semirestricted, and clean
   b. Unrestricted, clean, and dirty
   c. Unrestricted, clean, and restricted
   d. Unrestricted, semirestricted, and restricted

4. The locker room is a/an _____ area.
   a. Restricted
   b. Transitional
   c. Semirestricted
   d. None of the above

5. Only personnel in complete scrub attire, including hair cap, mask, and facial hair covering, are permitted in the _____ area.
   a. Restricted
   b. Unrestricted
   c. Semirestricted
   d. None of the above

6. The _____ core contains clean and sterile equipment and supplies.
   a. Clean
   b. Sterile
   c. Central
   d. Equipment

7. The primary design goal of the floor plan is to create a clear separation between _____ and _____ equipment.
   a. Sterile, clean
   b. Soiled, contaminated
   c. Soiled, clean
   d. Dirty, soiled

8. _____ in the surgical suite are stored in closed cabinets to keep them clean.
   a. Sterile supplies
   b. The computer and accessories
   c. Anesthesia drugs
   d. Anesthesia hoses and masks

9. The operating room table is adjustable for height, degree of tilt in all directions, orientation in the room, articular breaks, and _____.
   a. Patient weight capacity
   b. Ability to be used for transport
   c. Safety features
   d. Length

10. The back table is a large, stainless steel table on which all instruments, supplies, and equipment needed for surgery are arranged, except for those needed for:
    a. Immediate use
    b. Delivery of anesthesia
    c. Later in the case
    d. Suturing

CASE STUDIES

1. *Read the following case study and, using the information given, create a line chain of command for the facility.*

   You have been recently hired at your local hospital. Mr. Hall is the Chief Operations Officer (COO). He has just been hired. He asks you if you could show him the chain of command for your area of surgical services. Because you work in a very small hospital, there are only two certified surgical technologists, you and one other scrub (Arlinda). Two nurses (Paul and Lydia) work in the OR.

   The charge nurse for your area is Mrs. Jones. She has worked at the hospital in this position for 25 years. The operating room staff educator's name is Abby. Mrs. Markus is the operating room nurse manager, and she reports to the director of perioperative services. His name is Mr. Smith. Mr. Smith reports to the vice president of patient care services, Mr. Zander.

   a. Design a linear chain of command including the name and titles of the individuals with the information provided.

2. *Your hospital has been bought out. They are looking for a new design for the operating room, and you have been chosen to be on the design team. They ask you to do the following:*

   a. Design an operating room.

b. Include all ancillary departments.

c. Include any other items you feel will enhance the department.

5 Supporting the Psychosocial Needs of the Patient

Student's Name _____

KEY TERMS

Write the definition for each term.

1. Anesthesia awareness: _____

2. Body image: _____

3. Maslow's hierarchy of human needs: _____

4. Patient-centered care: _____

5. Physiological: _____

6. Self-actualization: _____

SHORT ANSWERS

Provide a short answer for each question or statement.

1. What is the philosophy of Roger's patient-centered care?

_____

_____

2. What does Maslow's chart teach us about the needs of individuals?

_____

_____

3. Why would a patient feel a loss of security if he or she were about to undergo a surgical procedure?

_____

_____

4. Therapeutic supportive patient communication includes:

_____

_____

5. List effective ways of communicating with the elderly patient.

_____

_____

6. Explain developmental disability and how it affects communication.

_____

_____

7. What are some common fears of patients prior to surgery?

_____

_____

MATCHING

Define Maslow's triangular hierarchy with the correct definition and give an example of each.

1. _____ Sleep   a. Physiological

2. _____ Temperature   b. Protection

3. _____ Mobility   c. Relational

4. _____ Safety   d. Self-actualization

5. _____ Security

6. _____ Belonging

7. _____ Altered body image

8. _____ Achieving personal goals

9. _____ Elimination

10. _____ Respiration

11. _____ Love

12. _____ Nutrition

MATCHING

Match the appropriate developmental age groups to the following descriptions.

1. _____ Curious about their bodies, often insist on "helping" with their own care.

2. _____ The operating room is terrifying, there is a strong fear of the unknown, commonly view the hospital and OR as punishment.

3. _____ Very sensitive about body image, resistant to intrusion of privacy and physical exposure.

4. _____ Becomes extremely anxious and frustrated when separated from their primary care provider.

5. _____ Needs to be physically close to their caregivers, often accompanied to the OR by the primary care provider.

a.	Infant	birth to 18 months
b.	Toddler	19 months to 3 years
c.	Preschool	3 to 6 years
d.	School age	7 to 12 years
e.	Adolescent	13 to 18 years

MULTIPLE CHOICE

Choose the most correct answer for each question or statement.

1. According to Maslow's hierarchy of needs, the most basic of human needs are:
   a. Psychological
   b. Physiological
   c. Metabolic
   d. Pathological

2. Maslow's hierarchy of human needs is depicted as a triangular hierarchy in which the critical needs to preserve life are at the base levels, and other needs that create the rest of the hierarchy are:
   a. Emotional
   b. Social
   c. Spiritual fulfillment
   d. All the above

3. A patient's fear that he or she will not awaken from the anesthetic, or will feel pain while remaining paralyzed, is called:
   a. Anesthesia
   b. Anesthesia awareness
   c. Anesthesia provider
   d. Anesthetic agents

4. Fear of _____ during or after surgery is common among patients who are about to receive a general anesthetic or undergo radical cancer surgery.
   a. Pain
   b. Physical exposure
   c. Loss of control
   d. Death

5. Fear of _____ is a normal protective mechanism.
   a. Pain
   b. Disfigurement
   c. Loss of control
   d. Death

6. Patients undergoing radical or reconstructive surgery have realistic fears about:
   a. Pain
   b. Disfigurement
   c. Loss of control
   d. Death

7. When patients enter the health care system, they often feel a loss of personal rights and _____.
   a. Pain
   b. Disfigurement
   c. Control
   d. Death

8. The fear of _____ of the body is quite strong in many patients, especially adolescents.
   a. Pain exposure
   b. Physical exposure
   c. Control
   d. Death

9. _____ are powerful needs that determine sense of well-being through the acceptance and nurturing of others.
   a. Esteem
   b. Self-actualization
   c. Love and belonging
   d. Spiritual needs

10. Many patients are afraid that information about their health may not be held in confidence. This is a fear of:
    a. Loss of privacy
    b. Physical exposure
    c. Control
    d. Death

11. Patients often express their religious _____ while in the health care setting. _____ can be a major force for many patients and may even play an equal role in their well-being along with the surgical procedures they undergo.
    a. Love
    b. Belonging
    c. Self-actualization
    d. Faith

12. Maslow's model includes _____ and self-image because the perception we have of ourselves influences motivation and relationships, both social and personal.
    a. Self-esteem
    b. Feelings of acceptance
    c. Family needs
    d. Self-doubt

13. _____ is dependent not only on physical appearance but also on people's normal roles within their family and community.
    a. Self-esteem
    b. Feelings of acceptance
    c. Family needs
    d. Self-image

CASE STUDIES

1. *Read the following case study and answer the questions based on your knowledge of therapeutic communication and geriatric patients:*

You have been asked by the operating room (OR) supervisor to help transport an elderly patient to the pre-op holding area from her patient room. The patient was recently diagnosed with breast cancer. You enter the patient's room and introduce yourself. The following conversation ensues:

You: "Hello, sweetie. My name is Jane Smith, and I'm here to transport you to surgery today. Can you please tell me the name of your surgeon and the type of procedure you will be having today?"

Mrs. Smith: "Dr. Woods is my surgeon, and he is going to remove my cancer today."

You: "Could you be more specific, Mrs. Smith? Where is your cancer?"

Mrs. Smith: "The cancer is in my left breast. (pause) I'm worried about the surgery. My friend said that the procedure is very disfiguring."

You: "Many patients are afraid of surgery, Mrs. Smith."

Mrs. Smith: "I'm worried that I might die from the cancer if the doctor doesn't get it all out."

You: "Would you like to talk to someone about this before we go to surgery?"

Mrs. Smith: "No, I guess not. I'm ready to go."

You: "Okay, can I get you to scoot over to the OR stretcher for me?"

Now answer the following questions about this conversation:

a. Are you comfortable with the way this conversation has gone?

b. Was the conversation helpful in alleviating the patient's fear before you brought her to surgery?

c. Is the conversation you are having with the patient helpful or therapeutic?

d. Modify the conversation so that it becomes therapeutic for the patient. Change your responses above.

2. *Design a Maslow's hierarchy needs chart.*

a. Give an example of each area and how it pertains to the surgical patient.

b. How does the hierarchy relate to the CST during care of the surgical patient?

c. What happens if one area is not given the right attention at the right time?

Student's Name _____

KEY TERMS

Write the definition for each term.

1. ABO blood group _____

2. Acute illness _____

3. Benign _____

4. Chronic illness _____

5. Complete blood count (CBC) _____

6. Computed tomography (CT) _____

7. Contrast medium _____

8. Diastolic pressure _____

9. Differential count _____

10. Digital radiography _____

11. Doppler studies _____

12. Electrocardiography _____

13. Endoscopic procedures _____

14. Fluoroscopy _____

15. Hematocrit (Hct) _____

16. Hemoglobin (Hgb) _____

17. Imaging studies _____

18. Invasive procedure _____

19. Magnetic resonance imaging _____

20. Malignant _____

21. Mean arterial pressure (MAP) _____

22. Metastasis _____

23. Neoplasm _____

24. Nuclear medicine _____

25. Orthostatic (postural) blood pressure _____

26. Palpating _____

27. Partial thromboplastin time (PTT) _____

28. Positron emission tomography (PET) _____

29. Prothrombin time (PT) _____

30. Pulse pressure _____

31. Radioactive seed _____

32. Radionuclide or isotopes _____

33. Radiopaque _____

34. Sphygmomanometer _____

35. Staging _____

36. Systolic pressure _____

37. TNM classification system _____

38. Transcutaneous _____

39. Tumor marker _____

40. Vital signs _____

SHORT ANSWERS

Provide a short answer for each question or statement.

1. The vital signs include:

_____

_____

2. During surgery, why is it important to monitor vital signs?

_____

_____

3. What is the difference between acute and chronic illness? Give an example of each.

_____

_____

4. Name six different ways a patient's temperature might be taken?

a. _____

b. _____

c. _____

d. _____

e. _____

f. _____

5. Explain the three- or four-point scale used to report the strength of the pulse, as well as the terminology used to describe the pulse.

_____

_____

_____

_____

_____

6. Describe the technique for measuring the respiratory rate.

_____

_____

7. Describe the technique of evaluating the pulse using the associated terms and definitions.

_____

_____

_____

8. List the areas for measuring the pulse.

_____

_____

9. What can alter the respiratory rate?

_____

_____

10. What problems are associated with evaluation of a patient's blood pressure using a simple digital (automatic) sphygmomanometer?

_____

_____

_____

11. Blood pressure varies by age and is affected by various other normal physiological conditions including:

_____

_____

12. Important normal physiological factors that influence blood pressure include:

_____

_____

13. List the technique for taking the blood pressure.

_____

_____

14. List the common errors associated with blood pressure measurement.

_____

_____

15. The CBC is a basic test used to evaluate the type and percentage of normal components in the blood. What five components are tested?

_____

_____

_____

_____

16. Positively charged electrolytes are called *cations*. Which cations are routinely tested during a routine blood workup?

_____

_____

MATCHING

Match each term with the correct definition.

1. _____ A combination of x-ray and digital technology in which images are captured and translated to a flat panel screen that is visible in normal lighting.

2. _____ Is generated by high-frequency sound waves.

3. _____ Uses radiofrequency signals and multiple magnetic fields to produce a high-definition image.

4. _____ Uses the combined technologies of computed tomography and radioactive scanning.

5. _____ X-ray and computer technologies are combined to produce high-contrast cross-sectional images.

a. Computed tomography (CT)

b. Magnetic resource imaging (MRI)

c. Fluoroscopy

d. Positron emission tomography (PET)

e. Ultrasound

MATCHING

1. _____ A person's blood type.

2. _____ Is a basic test used to evaluate the type and percentage of normal components in the blood.

3. _____ The mechanism of blood clotting.

4. _____ Cations and anions.

5. _____ Includes blood glucose, carbon dioxide, creatinine, urea nitrogen, bicarbonate, and several important electrolytes.

a. Complete blood count

b. Metabolic panel

c. Coagulation test

d. Arterial blood gases

e. ABO groups

f. Electrolytes

MATCHING

Match the blood pressure technique with its error. You may use the same answer more than once.

1. _____ Pressing the stethoscope too hard on the artery.

2. _____ Cuff is too loose for the patient.

3. _____ Cuff is too small for the patient.

4. _____ Failure to wait longer than 2 minutes before retaking the blood pressure.

5. _____ Cuff is deflated too quickly.

6. _____ Cuff is deflated too slowly.

7. _____ Air escapes from the cuff even when the valve is closed.

8. _____ Stopping deflation and reinflating the cuff.

a. Faulty equipment

b. False high diastolic

c. False low diastolic

d. False low systolic

e. False high systolic and diastolic

MULTIPLE CHOICE

Choose the most correct answer to complete the question or statement.

1. The most basic form of clinical assessment is (a/an):
   a. CT scan
   b. Chest radiograph
   c. ECG
   d. Vital signs

2. The body requires a core (internal) temperature of approximately 99° F, or
   a. 37.2° C
   b. 38.2° C
   c. 40° C
   d. 42° C

3. Axillary temperature readings are _____ than oral measurements.
   a. 0.3° to 0.6° C higher
   b. 0.5° to 1° F lower
   c. 0.5° C and 1.5° C lower
   d. 0.6° C and 1.6° C higher

4. Which statement about the use of thermometers is true?
   a. Rectal thermometers are the preferred method for measuring temperature.
   b. You do not need to wash your hands after taking a patient's temperature with a forehead or skin thermometer because it is not an invasive procedure.
   c. The rectal method is preferred over the tympanic method.
   d. Tympanic thermometers have a single-use probe cover that is used to prevent cross-contamination of patients.

5. The normal pulse rate for an adult is _____.
   a. 40 to 60 beats per minute
   b. 60 to 100 beats per minute
   c. 75 to 110 beats per minute
   d. 80 to 120 beats per minute

6. The pulse range for an athlete is:
   a. 50 to 100 beats per minute
   b. 60 to 100 beats per minute
   c. 75 to 110 beats per minute
   d. 80 to 120 beats per minute

7. _____ provides detailed information about heart conduction.
   a. ECG
   b. EEG
   c. Blood pressure
   d. Oximetry

8. The basic metabolic panel includes all of the following, *except:*
   a. Blood glucose
   b. Carbon dioxide
   c. Creatinine
   d. Oxygen

9. _____ is performed to assess the functional ability of the coagulation sequence.
   a. Electrolyte testing
   b. ABO group testing
   c. PTT
   d. Measurement of ABG levels

10. Electrolytes include all the following, *except:*
    a. Sodium
    b. Carbonic acid
    c. Potassium
    d. Calcium

11. Hypocalcemia is caused from a deficiency of what electrolyte?
    a. Calcium
    b. Potassium
    c. Sodium
    d. None of the above

12. Hyponatremia is caused from a deficiency of what electrolyte?
    a. Calcium
    b. Potassium
    c. Sodium
    d. None of the above

13. Hypokalemia is caused from a deficiency of what electrolyte?
    a. Calcium
    b. Potassium
    c. Sodium
    d. None of the above

14. Urinalysis is performed to assess the body's overall health, with particular focus on the urinary tract; a simple screening is performed to check for different substances to include all, *except:*
    a. Albumin
    b. Glucose
    c. Magnesium
    d. Leukocytes

15. One of the tests used to detect the type of infection is the:
    a. Biopsy and aspiration
    b. Sensitivity and aspiration
    c. Culture and biopsy
    d. Culture and sensitivity

16. The surgical removal of a small portion of tissue is a(n):
    a. Needle or trocar biopsy
    b. Brush biopsy
    c. Excision
    d. Smear

17. Biopsy obtained by passing a small cylandrical brush is used to sweep a hollow lumen or cavity for cells?
    a. Needle or trocar biopsy
    b. Brush biopsy
    c. Excision
    d. Core biopsy

18. What is used to sweep a hollow lumen or cavity for cells?
    a. Needle or trocar biopsy
    b. Brush
    c. Excision
    d. Smear

19. A procedure in which a core sample of tissue is removed with a hollow needle or trocar in one or more locations of the suspected area is called:
    a. Needle or trocar biopsy
    b. Brush biopsy
    c. Excision
    d. Smear

20. Fluid for pathological examination may be removed and placed on a microscopic slide sprayed with a cell fixative.
    a. Needle or trocar biopsy
    b. Brush biopsy
    c. Aspiration biopsy
    d. Smear

21. A procedure in which tissue is removed and immediately placed in liquid nitrogen is called:
    a. Frozen section
    b. Brush biopsy
    c. Excision
    d. Smear

22. An abnormal growth of tissue that can be benign or malignant
    a. Malignant tumor
    b. Benign tumor
    c. Metastasis
    d. Neoplasm

23. What is composed of cells belonging to a single tissue type and does not spread to distant regions of the body?
    a. Malignant tumor
    b. Benign tumor
    c. Metastasis
    d. Neoplasm

24. New tumors may develop from these "seed" cells.
    a. Malignant tumor
    b. Benign tumor
    c. Metastasis
    d. Neoplasm

25. What is composed of disorganized tissue that exhibits uncontrolled growth?
    a. Malignant tumor
    b. Benign tumor
    c. Metastasis
    d. Neoplasm

26. The culture and sensitivity test is used to:
    a. Determine the presence of a foreign body in tissue
    b. Identify the exact microorganism and appropriate antibiotic to treat the infection.
    c. Detect an infectious agent
    d. Detect the presence of pus in a wound

27. A neoplasm:
    a. Is usually malignant
    b. Does not undergo histological change
    c. Is always benign
    d. Is any abnormal growth

28. Malignant tumors:
    a. Closely resemble the tissue or origin
    b. Release toxins that kill normal cells
    c. Capture nutrients from normal cells
    d. Are single tissue type

29. Metastasis is:
    a. The spread of a benign tumor into other tissues
    b. A tumor that is confined and does not infiltrate the tissue bed
    c. A tumor that exhibits organized growth patterns
    d. Often propagated by seed cells that break away from the tumor, which spreads to distant locations of the body

30. Magnetic resonance imaging (MRI) uses magnetic energy to detect structural tissue abnormalities. Which of the following can cause distortion of MRI imaging?
    a. Biomedical devices
    b. Tattoos containing metal-based dye
    c. Vascular clips
    d. All of the above

31. Which of the following is used during surgery to provide moving images to be seen in real-time?
    a. MRI
    b. PET scan
    c. Fluoroscopy
    d. X-ray

32. Which of the following WBC levels indicate infection?
    a. 5000
    b. 12,000
    c. 8000
    d. 10,000

CASE STUDIES

1. *You are asked to take the patient's vital signs. You can only find one blood pressure cuff. It is intended for normal adults. Your patient's BMI is 40 (morbidly obese).*

    a. How will this cuff affect the blood pressure reading?

37

Chapter 6 Diagnostic and Assessment Procedures

Copyright © 2022 Elsevier, Inc. All rights reserved.

b. Can you use this cuff as long as you document which size you used?

c. While the cuff is being inflated, it suddenly pops off the patient's arm. How should you proceed?

7 Environmental Hazards

Student's Name _____

Write the definition for each term.

1. Airborne transmission precautions: _____

2. Blood-borne pathogens: _____

3. Electrocution: _____

4. Electrosurgical unit: _____

5. Eschar: _____

6. Flammable: _____

7. Grounding: _____

8. Hypersensitivity: _____

9. Impedance (resistance): _____

10. Latex: _____

11. Neutral zone (no hands) technique: _____

12. Occupational exposure: _____

13. Oxiders: _____

14. Oxygen-enriched atmosphere (OEA): _____

15. Personal protective equipment: _____

16. Postexposure prophylaxis: _____

17. Risk: _____

18. Sharps: _____

19. Smoke plume: _____

20. Standard Precautions: _____

21. Transmission-based precautions: _____

22. Underwriters laboratories: _____

23. Volatile: _____

Provide a short answer for each question or statement.

1. What is the fire triangle? How do the components relate to each other?

   _____

   _____

2. What is a "source of ignition"?

   _____

   _____

3. What is a patient fire? What are the percentages of the most common locations where patient fires occur? What needs to be done to stop the profression of the fire?

   _____

   _____

4. List several fuels that are capable of causing surgical site fires and explain how to prevent them.

   _____

   _____

5. Name the common sources of ignition found in the operating room.

   _____

   _____

6. If a fire breaks out in the operating room, what three steps should be taken immediately to protect the patient and put out the fire?

   _____

   _____

7. What parts of a compressed gas cylinder should you inspect for safe operation?

   _____

   _____

8. Describe the recommended procedure for transporting compressed gas cylinders in the health care facility.

   _____

   _____

9. List the guidelines for storage of gas cylinders.

   _____

   _____

10. What is a Material Safety Data Sheet?

_____

_____

11. Why are Standard Precautions used in health care?

_____

_____

12. What diseases require airborne transmission precautions? Droplet precautions?

_____

_____

13. In the operating room, musculoskeletal injuries most often occur as a result of:

_____

_____

LABELING

Using the following triangle, draw in the three components required for fire. Under each of the three components, make a directory of the items specific to the operating room that fall into that section.

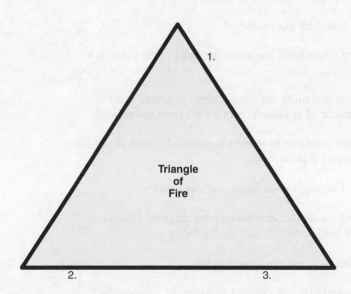

Triangle
of
Fire

1. _____

_____

_____

2. _____

   _____

   _____

3. _____

   _____

   _____

MATCHING

Determine whether each statement refers to ionizing radiation (a) or magnetic resonance imaging (b).

1. _____ A lead apron must be worn during fluoroscopy to prevent exposure
   to scatter radiation.

2. _____ Lead aprons must be stored flat or hung in a manner that prevents
   bending of the material.

3. _____ Remember that a lead apron protects only the areas of the body
   that are covered by the apron.

4. _____ The primary risk is the presence of metal, which can be drawn
   from its source and into the path of the powerful magnetic field.
   For this reason, absolutely no metal objects are permitted in the
   environment during this process.

5. _____ The eyes and hands are not protected.

6. _____ Cannot be used when there are metal implants in the patient or
   staff members.

7. _____ Those who must remain in the room during exposure must
   maintain a distance of at least 6 feet (1.8 m) from the patient.

8. _____ Neck shields are available to protect the thyroid, which is sensitive
   to radiation, during fluoroscopy.

9. _____ Cannot be used with personal items, such as jewelry.

10. _____ Nonsterile workers should step outside the range of exposure,
    either behind a lead screen or outside the room.

11. _____ Only plastic and titanium objects are safe.

12. _____ Lead glasses should be worn during exposure to a fluoroscope.

13. _____ The safest place to stand is at a right angle to the beam on the side
    of the radiograph machine or origin of the radiation beam.

a. Ionizing radiation

b. Magnetic resonance imaging

MATCHING

1. _____ ECRI

2. _____ CDC

3. _____ APIC

4. _____ EPA

5. _____ FDA

6. _____ TJC

7. _____ OSHA

8. _____ NIOSH

a. National Institute for Occupational Safety and Health

b. The Joint Commission

c. Occupational Safety and Health Administration

d. Centers for Disease Control and Prevention

e. Association for Professionals in Infection Control and Epidemiology

f. Agency for Healthcare Research and Quality

g. U.S. Environmental Protection Agency

h. U.S. Food and Drug Administration

MULTIPLE CHOICE

Choose the most correct answer to complete the question or statement.

1. Materials and substances that burn are called:
   a. Flammable
   b. Flame resistant
   c. Flame retardant
   d. High alert

2. Which of the following statements is true regarding the high fire risk in the operating room?
   a. Oxygen is heavier than air and settles on the floor.
   b. Oxygen is lighter than air and tends to float above the anesthesia machine.
   c. Oxygen may become confined in areas such as the groin and the axilla.
   d. When nitrous oxide decomposes in the presence of heat, oxygen molecules are produced, creating an oxygen-rich environment.

3. An environment that has a concentration of oxygen greater than 21% is called an:
   a. Oxygen-poor atmosphere
   b. Oxygen-enriched atmosphere
   c. Operating room oxygen
   d. Oxidizer

4. Which of the following are/is considered flammable?
   a. Endotracheal tubes
   b. Surgical drapes
   c. Fibrin glue
   d. All of the above

5. Which of the following are/is considered source(s) of ignition?
   a. Surgical drapes
   b. Laser
   c. Chlorhexidine
   d. Alcohol prepping solution

6. Which of the following acronyms should you remember if you are trying to put out a fire?
   a. PASS
   b. RACE
   c. RICE
   d. PAST

7. Compressed _____ is used as a power source for instruments, such as drills, saws, and other high-speed tools.
   a. Oxygen
   b. Argon
   c. Nitrogen
   d. Nitrous oxide

8. Which of the following compressed medical gases is used as an anesthetic gas?
   a. Oxygen
   b. Nitrous oxide
   c. Argon
   d. Carbon dioxide

9. Chemicals that are transferred from larger containers to smaller containers must be labeled with the exact information found on the _____.
   a. MSDS sheets
   b. Original container
   c. OSHA regulation sheets
   d. Manufacturer's directions

10. With regard to toxic chemicals in the operating room, which of the following statements is true?
    a. The cumulative effects can be much greater than the effects of any single exposure.
    b. Many of the chemicals are hazardous, but they usually produce only short-term effects.
    c. Guidelines for handling chemicals are designed to help in the development of risk strategies.
    d. Only the emergency department is required to maintain MSDS for chemicals.

11. Nonresistant materials include:
    a. Metal
    b. Water
    c. Human body
    d. All of the above
    e. None of the above

12. TB is a type of _____ transmission.
    a. Bloodborne
    b. Airborne
    c. Contact
    d. Standard

13. Rubella is a type of _____ transmission.
    a. Bloodborne
    b. Airborne
    c. Contact
    d. Standard

14. Influenza is a type of _____ transmission.
    a. Droplet
    b. Bloodborne
    c. Contact
    d. Standard

15. _____ is a naturally occurring sap obtained from rubber trees.
    a. OPA
    b. Radiation
    c. Latex
    d. None of the above

16. Scaling, drying, and cracks in skin are symptoms of what type of allergic skin reaction?
    a. Contact dermatitis (nonallergic)
    b. Allergic contact dermatitis
    c. Natural rubber latex allergy
    d. Hypersensitivity

17. _____ causes dermatitis on contact with the object.
    a. Contact dermatitis (nonallergic)
    b. Allergic contact dermatitis
    c. Natural rubber latex allergy
    d. Hypersensitivity

18. _____ is the amount of physical effort needed to perform a task, such as moving an object.
    a. Posture
    b. Repetitive motion
    c. Exertion
    d. Contact stress

19. _____ is a critical component of musculo-skeletal stress.
    a. Posture
    b. Repetitive motion
    c. Exertion
    d. Contact stress

20. _____ places stress on tendons and muscles.
    a. Posture
    b. Repetitive motion
    c. Exertion
    d. Contact stress

21. When _____, keep the object close to your body.
    a. Lifting
    b. Pushing and pulling
    c. Bending
    d. Standing

22. When _____, place one foot behind the other, with back foot braced comfortably.
    a. Lifting
    b. Pushing and pulling
    c. Bending
    d. Standing

CASE STUDIES

1. *Read the following case study and answer the questions based on your knowledge of fire in the operating room:*

   You are scrubbed in for an endoscopic procedure. The surgeon has disconnected the light cord from the endoscope and placed it on the surgical drapes without turning it off.

   a. What can you say to the surgeon about safety related to this?

   b. What is your own role here?

2. *Read the following case study and answer the questions based on your knowledge of fire in the operating room:*

   You are searching the OR suite for something that smells as if it is overheating. You see that a C-arm fluoroscopy machine is plugged into the wall. While you are calling the radiology department to come and check out the machine, it bursts into flames.

   a. Using the acronym RACE, describe the actions you will take.

   R _____

   A _____

   C _____

   E _____

45

8 Microbes and the Process of Infection

Student's Name _____

KEY TERMS

Write the definition for each term.

1. Aerobes: _____

2. Aerosol droplets: _____

3. Anaerobes: _____

4. Bioburden: _____

5. Contaminated: _____

6. Cross-contamination: _____

7. Culture: _____

8. Diffusion: _____

9. Direct transmission: _____

10. Droplet nuclei: _____

11. Endospore: _____

12. Entry site: _____

13. Fomite: _____

14. Infection: _____

15. Inflammation: _____

16. Necrosis: _____

17. Nosocomial infection: _____

18. Opportunistic infection: _____

19. Pathogen: _____

20. Prion: _____

21. Resident microorganism: _____

22. Sterile: _____

23. Suppurative: _____

24. Vector: _____

25. Virion: _____

26. Virulence: _____

SHORT ANSWERS

Provide a short answer for each question or statement.

1. List the tools for identifying microbes and give an example of each.

_____

_____

2. A surgical site infection may start as an abscess. What exactly is an abscess?

_____

_____

3. Bacteria that cause infection are called pathogenic. List common pathogenic microbes.

_____

_____

4. List the most important methods of disease prevention in the health care facility.

_____

_____

5. List physiological risks for surgical site infection.

_____

_____

6. Describe and provide examples of nosocomial infection.

_____

_____

MATCHING

Match the microbe with the correct definition and example.

1. _____ an organism lives on or within another organism (the host) and gains an advantage at the expense of that organism.

2. _____ one organism uses another to meet its physiological needs but causes no harm to the host. For example, the normal human intestinal tract contains many different types of bacteria, such as *Escherichia coli,* that are essential for metabolism.

3. _____ only about 3% to 5% of all microbes are pathogenic. However, nonpathogenic microbes (those that do not usually cause disease) that live in and on the body can become pathogenic under certain conditions.

4. _____ each of the organisms benefits from their relationship in the environment. For example, *Staphylococcus aureus* inhabits normal, healthy skin.

a. Commensalism

b. Mutualism

c. Parasitism

d. Opportunistic organisms

MATCHING

Match the disease transmission with the proper term.

1. _____ *Staphylococcus aureus*

2. _____ Talking, coughing, or sneezing

3. _____ Food

4. _____ Blood-borne pathogens

5. _____ Vector

a. Direct contact

b. Airborne transmission

c. Transmission by body fluids

d. Oral transmission (ingestion)

e. Fly

MATCHING

1. _____ Straight or curved rod shaped bacteria, which can occur singly or in pairs, chains or filaments.

2. _____ Comma-shaped bacteria.

3. _____ Single spherical-shaped bacteria.

4. _____ Curved or spiral-shaped bacteria that may be coiled or loosely curved.

5. _____ Spherical-shaped bacteria.

6. _____ Spherical-shaped bacteria in groups of four or in clusters.

7. _____ A pair of spherical-shaped bacteria.

8. _____ A chain of spherical-shaped bacteria.

a. *Vibrio*

b. *Cocci*

c. *Spirochetes*

d. *Staphylococci*

e. *Streptococci*

f. *Bacilli*

g. *Diplococci*

h. *Micrococci*

MULTIPLE CHOICE

Choose the most correct answer to complete the question or statement.

1. Virology is the study of:
   a. Disease mechanisms, diagnosis, and treatment
   b. Bacteria
   c. Microbes
   d. Viruses

2. Which of the following is *not* a characteristic of eukaryotic cells?
   a. Multicellular
   b. Double-layer membrane
   c. Cell membrane
   d. Include bacteria and Archaea

3. The primary structural difference between the prokaryote and eukaryote is:
   a. Prokaryotes are more like human cells.
   b. Prokaryotes have a semipermeable cell membrane.
   c. Prokaryotes have no distinct nucleus.
   d. Eukaryotes are not pathogenic.

4. The _____ protects the cell from drying and provides resistance to chemicals and invasion by viruses.
   a. Cell wall
   b. Capsule
   c. Cell membrane
   d. Spores

5. The _____ is also called the slime layer.
   a. Cell wall
   b. Cell membrane
   c. Outside layer of the nucleus
   d. Capsule

6. _____ is a process in which particles are engulfed.
   a. Phagocytosis
   b. Pinocytosis
   c. Active transport
   d. Endocytosis

7. The human intestinal tract contains many different types of bacteria, such as *Escherichia coli,* which are essential for digestion. This is an example of:
   a. Mutualism
   b. Parasitism
   c. Symbiosis
   d. Commensalism

8. What is the most effective way of controlling cross-contamination in the health facility environment?
   a. Handwashing
   b. Sterilization of instruments before surgery
   c. Keeping patient rooms clean
   d. Providing lockers for each employee

9. In the _____ phase, symptoms begin to appear.
   a. Incubation
   b. Prodromal phase
   c. Acute phase
   d. Convalescence

10. In the _____ phase, the organism is at its most potent.
    a. Incubation
    b. Prodromal phase
    c. Acute phase
    d. Convalescence

11. In the _____ phase, the pathogens actively replicate.
    a. Incubation
    b. Prodromal phase
    c. Acute phase
    d. Convalescence

12. During the _____ phase, proliferation of the infectious organism slows and symptoms subside.
    a. Incubation
    b. Prodromal phase
    c. Acute phase
    d. Convalescence

13. The prion diseases are very significant in the surgical setting because:
    a. They spread rapidly
    b. All surgical patients are at risk
    c. It is impossible to know who is a carrier
    d. They are resistant to all usual methods of destruction

14. Skin and mucous membrane are considered the first line of defense against disease because:
    a. Skin can be sterilized using disinfectants
    b. Once the skin is broken, infection can develop
    c. Skin contains many blood vessels
    d. Skin is very strong

15. Which surgical wound is associated with a higher risk of infection in the postoperative patient?
    a. Clean
    b. Clean-contaminated
    c. Contaminated
    d. All the above

16. The cardinal signs of inflammation are:
    a. Heat, redness, pain, swelling
    b. Pus, pain, redness, swelling
    c. Heat, pus, fever, pain
    d. Both A and C

49

17. Surgical site infection begins when a pathogenic or nonpathogenic microorganism colonizes sterile tissues. This can be caused by:
    a. Contamination of the tissues, such as a ruptured bowel or a traumatic wound caused by a foreign object
    b. External contamination of the wound during convalescence
    c. Poor surgical technique
    d. All of the above

18. Bacteria that causes infection is called:
    a. Contagious
    b. Toxic
    c. Pyogenic
    d. None of the above

19. Surgical site infection represents:
    a. The greatest cause of hospital-acquired infection
    b. The second most common cause of hospital-acquired infection
    c. The most avoidable cause of hospital-acquired infection
    d. The main reason for a hospital to lose accreditation

20. Bacteria require basic elemental nutrients, except:
    a. Oxygen
    b. Sulfur
    c. Water
    d. Carbon

21. All of the following are Gram-positive bacteria, except:
    a. Staphylococcus epidermidis
    b. Streptococcus Pyogenes
    c. Gonorrhea
    d. Streptococcus Pneumoniae

22. A _____ is a nonliving infectious agent that ranges in size from 10 to 300 nm.
    a. Bacterium
    b. Virus
    c. Fungi
    d. Prion

23. The _____ is a unique pathogenic substance.
    a. Bacteria
    b. Virus
    c. Fungi
    d. Prion

24. _____ are found worldwide on living organic substances, in water, and in soil.
    a. Bacteria
    b. Viruses
    c. Fungi
    d. Prions

25. _____ are a group of single-cell eukaryotic organisms.
    a. Protozoa
    b. Virus
    c. Fungi
    d. Algae

26. _____ are eukaryotes that belong to the plant kingdom; they include sponges and seaweed.
    a. Protozoa
    b. Virus
    c. Fungi
    d. Algae

27. _____ exists from the time of birth.
    a. Innate immunity
    b. Adaptive immunity

28. _____ conferred through exposure to a specific substance or microbe called an antigen.
    a. Innate immunity
    b. Adaptive immunity

29. _____ develops when the body receives the specific disease antibodies from an outside source.
    a. Active immunity
    b. Passive immunity
    c. Vaccination
    d. Hypersensitivity

30. Immune response to a substance is referred to as:
    a. Active
    b. Passive
    c. Vaccines
    d. Hypersensitivity

31. _____ is a process mediated by the immune system.
    a. True allergy
    b. Passive
    c. Vaccines
    d. Hypersensitivity

32. In certain diseases, the body does not recognize "self." This is known as _____.
    a. True allergy
    b. Autoimmunity
    c. Vaccines
    d. Hypersensitivity

33. There are two types of true allergic reactions:
    a. Immediate and reaction
    b. Reaction and delayed
    c. Delayed and immediate
    d. Immediate and true

34. The most widespread cause of surgical site infection is:
    a. *Streptococcus pyogens*
    b. *Staphylococcus epidermidis*
    c. *Staphylococcus aureus*
    d. *Pseudomonas aeruginosa*

35. The resident bacteria of the GI tract that are the most common cause of urinary tract infections are:
    a. *Staphylococcus epidermis*
    b. *Escherichia coli*
    c. *Neisseria gonorrhoeae*
    d. *Pseudomonas aeruginosa*

36. Spore-forming anaerobic bacterium that causes rapid tissue death in deep sounds deprived of oxygen causing gas gangrene is:
    a. *Salmonella typhi*
    b. *Escherichia coli*
    c. *Clostridium tetani*
    d. *Clostridium perfringens*

37. Spore-forming bacteria that cause severe diarrhea are:
    a. *Clostridium difficile*
    b. *Clostridium perfringens*
    c. *Salmonella typhi*
    d. *Salmonella enterica*

38. A virulent form of *staphylococcus* that is mainly transmitted by direct contact with hands, equipment, and supplies is:
    a. *Escherichia coli*
    b. *Clostridium difficele*
    c. *Pseudomonas aeruginosa*
    d. Methicillin-resistant *staphylococcus aureus and epidermis*

CASE STUDIES

1. *Read the following case study and answer the questions based on your knowledge of microbiology.*

   You are a new surgical technologist setting up for a craniotomy. You are opening your supplies to get ready to set up for the procedure. You have just been informed that the patient is undergoing a brain biopsy for suspected Creutzfeldt-Jakob disease. You recall learning about prions in your microbiology class. What should you do?

9 Sterile Technique and Infection Control

Student's Name _____

KEY TERMS

Write the definition for each term.

1. Antiseptic: _____

2. Chemical barrier: _____

3. Containment and confinement: _____

4. Contaminated: _____

5. Contamination: _____

6. Double gloving: _____

7. Disinfection: _____

8. Gross contamination: _____

9. Hand hygiene: _____

10. Handwashing: _____

11. Hands-free technique: _____

12. Instructions for use (IFU): _____

13. Laminar air flow: _____

14. Neutral zone: _____

15. No-touch technique: _____

16. Nonsterile: _____

17. Nonsterile team members: _____

18. Physical barrier: _____

19. Postexposure prophylaxis (PEP): _____

20. PPE: _____

21. Sharps: _____

22. Squames: _____

23. Sterile field: _____

24. Sterile item: _____

25. Sterility: _____

26. Strike-through contamination: _____

27. Surgical conscience: _____

28. Surgical hand antisepsis: _____

29. Surgical scrub: _____

30. Surgical site infection (SSI): _____

31. Surgical wound: _____

SHORT ANSWERS

Provide a short answer for each question or statement.

1. List examples of hazardous medical waste materials.

   _____

   _____

   _____

   _____

2. Where is the sterile field? What is the center of the sterile field?

   _____

   _____

3. Sterile objects are contained or confined to create barriers to avoid contact with _____ areas or objects.

4. What should be done before opening any sterile packages?

   _____

   _____

   _____

5. The primary purpose of shoe covers is to _____.

6. _____, _____, and _____ are the three types of hand hygiene practiced in the operating room.

7. Masks must be worn in all restricted areas of the operating room. They should not be worn around the neck *at any time* because _____

   _____

   _____

Chapter **9** **Sterile Technique and Infection Control**

8. Home-laundered head caps are not sanctioned by any infection control agency because _____

_____

_____

9. What are the two methods for performing surgical hand antisepsis? _____

_____

_____

10. Sterile gowning and gloving takes place immediately after _____

_____

_____

11. The sterile towel, gown, and gloves should be opened on a clean surface away from where sterile instruments and

other equipment have been opened to prevent _____

_____

_____

12. Describe the purpose of good hand hygiene and why it is essential for health care professionals. _____

_____

_____

13. Double gloving is perferred over single gloving because _____

_____

_____

14. Closed gloving technique is used when _____

_____

_____

15. Open gloving technique is used for _____

_____

_____

16. When gloving another person, you should open the glove, grasp the upper edges, and offer it with the palm of the

glove facing _____

_____

_____

17. If a surgical team member contaminates their glove during surgery, the circulator will remove it. This is done by

offering the contaminated hand with the palm facing _____

_____

_____

MATCHING

Match each term with the correct definition.

1. _____ are made of a lint-free synthetic material that is woven loosely enough to allow the breath to pass through effectively but tightly enough to filter 99% of particles of 5 micrograms or larger.

2. _____ are often worn by nonsterile perioperative personnel, for comfort and to prevent contamination of the surgical field through bacterial shedding from the arms.

3. _____ of any kind is a potential source of pathogens.

4. _____ are worn to reduce contamination of the surgical field by loose hair and dandruff from the scalp.

5. Perioperative personnel should wear _____ that are comfortable and easy to keep clean and that protect the wearer against foot injury.

6. _____ are worn any time surgical staff leave the department temporarily.

7. OSHA mandates the use of _____ as part of its blood-borne pathogen standard to protect workers exposed to splashing and splatter of blood and other body fluids.

8. The _____ is designed to prevent the shedding of skin particles and hair into the environment and to protect the wearer from contact with soil and body fluids.

a. Protective eyewear/face shield

b. Head coverings

c. Jewelry

d. Scrub suit

e. Cover gowns/Lab coats

f. Nonsterile cover jacket

g. Masks

h. Shoes and covers

MATCHING

Match each term with the correct transmission precautions.

_____ 1. C-Difficile

_____ 2. Measles

_____ 3. Haemophilius influenzae type B

_____ 4. Herpes

_____ 5. HIV

_____ 6. Varicella

_____ 7. Impetigo

_____ 8. Nisseria meningitidis

_____ 9. MRSA

_____ 10. Streptococcal pharyngitis

_____ 11. Abscess

_____ 12. Rubella

_____ 13. HBV

a. Airborne transmission precautions

b. Blood-borne transmission precautions

c. Droplet transmission precautions

d. Contact transmission precautions

MATCHING

Match each area with the required air pressure that is required in the following areas.

_____ 1. Clean work room   a. Positive

_____ 2. Soiled work room   b. Negative

_____ 3. Sterile processing clean work room

_____ 4. Sterile processing decontamination

_____ 5. Operating room

_____ 6. Sterile storage rom

MULTIPLE CHOICE

Choose the most correct answer to the question or statement.

1. Which of the following is contamination occuring when fluid from a nonsterile surface penetrates the protective wrapper of a sterile item?
   a. tear in kimguard wrapper
   b. safety seal missing
   c. tear in plastic outerwrap
   d. strike-through

2. After an item has been sterilized, its sterility is maintained by:
   a. Surgical technologists
   b. Asepsis
   c. Decontamination
   d. Aseptic technique

3. The ethical and professional motivation that regulates a professional's behavior regarding disease transmission is known as:
   a. Tort
   b. Surgical law
   c. Surgical conscience
   d. Asepsis

4. A scrub suit must be changed if it:
   a. Is contaminated by blood or body fluid
   b. Comes in contact with the patient
   c. Comes in contact with any nonsterile item

5. Long-sleeved cover jackets are worn in the OR by the:
   a. Surgeon
   b. Scrub
   c. Circulator
   d. All of the above

6. At the end of the shift, the surgical technologist may place the scrub suit in his or her locker if:
   a. It is unsoiled
   b. It does not have gross contaminants on it
   c. The surgical technologist has worked less than 8 hours in it
   d. The surgical technologist must never place the scrub suit in their locker at the end of a shift

7. When changing from street clothes to a scrub suit for entering the operating room, the surgical technologist puts on which of the following items first?
   a. Scrub suit
   b. Shoe covers
   c. Cover jacket
   d. Mask

8. The term for the area under the fingernails is:
   a. Sublingual
   b. Subungual
   c. Buccal
   d. Ungal

9. In the surgical scrub, which of the following comes first?
   a. Scrubbing the forearms
   b. Scrubbing the fingers
   c. Remove debris from under the nail beds
   d. Applying the soap from fingers to elbows to "wash" the hands and arms

10. The surgical scrub extends to:
    a. 2 inches above the elbows
    b. The elbows
    c. Just below the elbows

11. When sterile supplies have been opened, the sterile setup is vulnerable to contamination. Once the sterile supplies have been opened, (select all that apply):
    a. They remain sterile for one hour
    b. You must tape the OR door closed
    c. They remain sterile for two hours
    d. They must be continuously monitored to ensure sterility

12. _____ is a way of making decisions and acting on proven methods.
    a. Evidence-based practice
    b. Surgical conscience
    c. Asepsis
    d. Aseptic technique

13. _____ is based on surgical conscience: that is, the ethical and professional motivation that regulates a professional's behaviors regarding disease transmission.
    a. Evidence-based practice
    b. Law
    c. Asepsis
    d. Aseptic technique

14. _____ occurs when the surgeon's gloved hand accidentally touches the nonsterile edge of the surgical drape.
    a. Contamination
    b. A surgical error
    c. Antisepsis
    d. Aseptic technique

15. The _____ is worn by both sterile and nonsterile surgical personnel in the perioperative environment.
    a. Scrub suit
    b. Body lotion
    c. Leather shoes
    d. Lab coat

16. At the close of the case, gown and gloves are removed:
    a. By pulling gloves off first
    b. By removing the gown first and then gloves
    c. By breaking all the ties with gloved hands after removing gloves
    d. By pulling from the back

17. Before opening a sterile pack, the scrub should also check the outside package for the:
    a. Right size
    b. Integrity
    c. Right wrap
    d. Colored tape

18. What operating room furniture should the large pack be placed on before opening?
    a. Ring stand
    b. Mayo stand
    c. Back table
    d. Prep stand

19. What operating room furniture should the instrument tray be placed on prior to opening?
    a. Ring stand
    b. Mayo stand
    c. Back table
    d. Prep stand

20. What operating room furniture should the basin set be placed on before opening?
    a. Ring stand
    b. Mayo stand
    c. Back table
    d. Prep stand

21. Items wrapped in _____ are delivered directly to the scrub by grasping the top edges of the wrapper and peeling the wrapper apart to reveal the sterile item.
    a. Sterile wrap
    b. Sealed pouches
    c. Sealed wrap
    d. Original package

22. What color is a biohazard bag?
    a. Clear
    b. Blue
    c. Red
    d. Yellow

23. The relative humidity of the operating room is within what range?
    a. 25%–65%
    b. 30%–70%
    c. 20%–60%
    d. 20%–70%

24. The recommended air exchanges per hour in the operating room is:
    a. 20–25
    b. 25–30
    c. 30–35
    d. 35–40

25. The range of temperature in the operating room is:
    a. 60–70 degrees F
    b. 65–70 degrees F
    c. 60–65 degrees F
    d. 68–75 degrees F

26. Unidirectional ultra-clean delivery system directing air away from the sterile field creating a "curtain" of air around the sterile field is called:
   a. Negative pressure
   b. Positive pressure
   c. Laminar air flow
   d. Scavenging system

27. Which of the following would require use of ethyl or isopropyl alcohol combined with skin emollients?
   a. Hand hygiene
   b. Surgical scrub
   c. Surgical rub

28. Which of the following would require use of a sterile brush?
   a. Hand hygiene
   b. Surgical scrub
   c. Surgical rub

CASE STUDIES

1. *You are about to begin clinicals and your instructor informed you one of the new students from another program accidently went to a restricted area of the department where she works. Your instructor has now asked you to name all of the zones of the operating room and their associated areas by function as well as describe the required attire for each of the zones.*

10 Decontamination, Sterilization, and Disinfection

Student's Name _____

<u>**KEY TERMS**</u>

Write the definition for each term.

1. Antiseptic _____

2. Antisepsis _____

3. Bactericidal _____

4. Bacteriostatic _____

5. Bioburden: _____

6. Biofilm _____

7. Biological indicators _____

8. Bowie Dick test _____

9. Case cart system _____

10. Cavitation _____

11. Central processing technician _____

12. Chemical indicator _____

13. Chemial sterilization _____

14. –cidal _____

15. Clean _____

16. Cleaning _____

17. Contaminated _____

18. Decontamination _____

19. Detergent _____

20. Disinfection _____

21. Enzymatic cleaner _____

22. Ethylene oxide (EO) _____

23. Event-related sterility _____

24. Exposure time _____

25. Fungicidal _____

26. Gas plasma sterilization _____

27. Germicidal _____

28. Gravity displacement sterilizer _____

29. High-level disinfection (HLD) _____

30. High-vacuum sterilizer _____

31. Cobalt-60 radiation _____

32. Inanimate _____

33. Implant _____

34. Immediate-use sterilization _____

35. Material Safety Data Sheets _____

36. Medical device _____

37. Noncritical items _____

38. Nonwoven _____

39. Peracetic acid _____

40. Personal protective equipment (PPE) _____

41. Physical monitor _____

42. Prion _____

43. Reposable _____

44. Reprocessing _____

45. Reusable _____

46. Sanitation _____

47. Sharps _____

48. Single-use items _____

49. Spaulding system _____

50. Sporicidal _____

51. Sterile processing department _____

52. Sterilization _____

53. Terminal cleaning _____

54. Turnover _____

55. Ultrasonic cleaner _____

56. Viricidal _____

57. Washer-sterilizer/decontaminator _____

58. Woven wrappers _____

SHORT ANSWERS

Provide a short answer for each question or statement.

1. Before the washer-sanitizer cycle is finished, the instruments are considered _____. What is the purpose of the washer-sterilizer?

_____

_____

_____

2. After the instruments are taken to the clean assembly area, what are the next steps for?

_____

_____

_____

3. Items with a lumen should have a small amount of _____ flushed through them immediately before sterilization.

_____

_____

MATCHING

Match each term with the correct definition. Some terms may be used more than once.

1. _____ Provides recommended practices and technical information for U.S. medical professions.

2. _____ Accreditation agency for all health care organizations in the United States.

3. _____ Professional association for perioperative nurses.

4. _____ An organization for which standards are developed with the support of the U.S. Food and Drug Administration.

5. _____ Agency of the federal government that provides research and protocols in all areas of public health.

6. _____ Organization that oversees compliance with environmental and patient safety regulations.

a. AAMI

b. AORN

c. CDC

d. TJC

MULTIPLE CHOICE

Choose the most correct answer to complete the question.

1. _____ is a chemical used to remove microorganisms on tissue.
   a. An antiseptic
   b. A disinfectant
   c. Sterilization
   d. All of the above

2. The system that assigns a patient care device a risk category for reprocessing on the specific regions of the body where the device is used is the _____ system.
   a. Spaulding
   b. Sterilization
   c. Dewey
   d. Maslow

3. Which of the following body tissues presents a high risk in the Spaulding system?
   a. Hands
   b. Intact skin
   c. Vascular system
   d. Mucosal membranes

4. _____ is a skilled, certified profession requiring expertise in the science and practice of materials management, decontamination, and sterilization.
   a. Perioperative nursing
   b. Anesthesiology
   c. Central processing technician
   d. Certified nurse's aides

5. The _____ is used to transport sterile and nonsterile instruments and equipment to and from the main operating room area.
   a. Crash cart
   b. Elevator
   c. Case cart

6. The washer-sterilizer or washer-disinfector is used to process all instruments that can tolerate
   a. Heat
   b. Water turbulence and high-pressure steam
   c. Strong disinfectant
   d. Cold solutions

7. After cleaning and disinfection, instruments are _____ to ensure smooth mechanical action.
   a. Unratcheted
   b. Lubricated
   c. Disinfected
   d. Wiped down with alcohol

8. Instruments that have _____ must be disassembled before cleaning and sterilization.
   a. Removable parts
   b. Ratchets
   c. Sharp edges
   d. Blades

9. Instrument trays have a perforated bottom so that:
   a. Steam can circulate up through the tray and adequately cover all surfaces of the instruments.
   b. They are easier for the surgical team to handle.
   c. The instruments are easily put into sets by central processing.
   d. The towels in the instrument sets cannot be damaged by the steam.

10. Which of the following statements is *not* true regarding the use of peel pouches?
    a. Items wrapped in peel pouches must not be placed inside an instrument tray.
    b. Double pouches are unnecessary and may prevent sterilization of the item.
    c. The item in the pouch should clear the seal by at least 1 inch.
    d. Peel pouches are intended for items such as bone rongeurs, rasps, and multiple instruments.

11. Which type of sterilization method requires an aeration?
    a. Steam
    b. Steam under pressure
    c. Ethylene oxide
    d. Gas plasma

12. Which of the following sterlization methods cloth or cellulose cannot be used and it requires items that are going to be sterilized to be clean and dry?
    a. Vaporized hydrogen peroxide
    b. Flash
    c. Ethylene oxide
    d. Steam

13. Which of the following high-level disinfectants could also be used as a sterilizing agent?
    a. Gas plasma
    b. Peracetic acid
    c. Glutaraldehyde
    d. Steam

14. The following are high-level disinfection semi-critical items, except:
    a. Operating room table and accessories
    b. Respiratory therapy equipment
    c. Bronchoscopes
    d. Anesthesia equipment

15. The following are low-level disinfection noncritical items, *except:*
    a. Stethoscopes
    b. Furniture in the surgical suite
    c. Bronchoscopes
    d. Blood pressure cuffs

16. Which is the cleaning process that removes debris from instruments in a process called cavitation?
    a. Cobalt-60
    b. Peracetic acid
    c. Ultrasonic
    d. Hydrogen peroxide

17. What is the exposure time for a wrapped tray of instruments at 250 degrees F?
    a. 15 minutes
    b. 20 minutes
    c. 30 minutes
    d. 45 minutes

18. What is the minimum exposure time for a wrapped tray of instruments at 270 degrees F?
    a. 15
    b. 20
    c. 30
    d. 45

19. Which is used to monitor air in the chamber of high-vacuum sterilizers?
    a. Bowie Dick
    b. Chemical indicator
    c. Mechanical indicator
    d. External chemical indicator

20. Which is the bacteria used to monitor steam sterilization effectiveness?
    a. *Bacillus subtilis*
    b. *Geobacillus stearothermophilis*
    c. *Stearothermophilius bacillus*
    d. *Geobacillus subtilis*

21. During surgery, if there is blood spilled on the floor in the operating room, what should the circulator do?
    a. Wipe and clean the area with a hospital-grade disinfectant
    b. Call housekeeping
    c. Cover it
    d. Do nothing

22. Routine cleaning of the operating room at the close of surgery each day is:
    a. Environmental
    b. Decontamination
    c. Damp dusting
    d. Terminal

CASE STUDIES

1. *Read the following case study and answer the following questions.*

   You are working in an ambulatory ophthalmic surgery center. You have a dual role at the facility—you scrub in surgery and also process and sterilize the instruments. Some of Dr. Smith's patients have developed some postoperative complications after cataract surgery recently.

   a. What is the most probable condition that has occured?

b. What are the causative factors that can contribute to this condition?

c. List AAMI guidelines for processing of ophthalmic instruments to prevent TASS.

11 Surgical Instruments

Student's Name _____

KEY TERMS

Write the definition for each term.

1. Alloy: _____

2. Anastomosis: _____

   _____

3. Box lock: _____

4. Chisel: _____

5. Curettage: _____

6. Dilator: _____

7. Double-action rongeur: _____

8. Elevator: _____

9. Gouge: _____

10. Hemostat: _____

11. Rongeur: _____

12. Resection: _____

    _____

13. Serosa: _____

14. Shank: _____

15. Single-action rongeur: _____

16. Tenaculum: _____

LABELING

Label the following diagram of a locking clamp.

1. _____

2. _____

3. _____

4. _____

5. _____

MATCHING

Match each instrument with its classification or function.

1. _____ Crile

2. _____ Allis

3. _____ Babcock

4. _____ Adson

5. _____ Poole

6. _____ Chisel

7. _____ Baumgartner

8. _____ Key

9. _____ Curved Mayo

10. _____ Sarot

11. _____ Kelly

12. _____ Gelpi

13. _____ Leksell

14. _____ Cobb

15. _____ Senn

16. _____ Weitlaner

17. _____ Pituitary

18. _____ Harrington

a. Cutting

b. Clamping/grasping

c. Hemostatic clamp

d. Suturing/needle holder

e. Dilator

f. Handheld retractor

g. Stapling

h. Hemostatic clip

i. Rongeur

j. Self-retaining retractor

k. Probing

l. Periosteal elevator

m. Tissue forcep

n. Atraumatic clamp

o. Filing bone

p. Suction

q. Scraping tissue or bone

19. _____ GIA

20. _____ Russian

21. _____ Osteotome

22. _____ Israel

23. _____ Yankauer

24. _____ Mayo-Hegar

25. _____ Metzenbaum

26. _____ Curette

27. _____ Kerrison

28. _____ Duval

29. _____ Mosquito

30. _____ Debakey

31. _____ Richardson

32. _____ Kocher Oschner

33. _____ Clip applier

34. _____ Balfour

35. _____ Frazier

36. _____ Deaver

37. _____ LDS

38. _____ Rasp

39. _____ Gigli

40. _____ Rake

MATCHING

Match each stapler with the name and function.

1. _____ Performs end-to-end intestinal resection and anastomosis.

2. _____ Right angle used to fit around deep structures for resection and anastomosis.

3. _____ Used for linear side-to-side and end-to-side anastomosis.

4. _____ Suture line is placed around the full circumference of a tubular structure.

5. _____ Places a single line of staples across skin edges.

6. _____ V-shaped staples used to occlude vessels or ducts.

a. Skin stapler

b. GIA Gastrointestinal anastomosis stapler

c. EEA End-to-end anastomosis stapler

d. TA Transverse anastomosis stapler

e. Purse-string stapler

f. Hemostatic clips

MATCHING

Match the correct knife handle with the correct blade.

1. _____ Microblade

2. _____ # 10

3. _____ # 11

4. _____ # 12

5. _____ # 15

6. _____ # 20

7. _____ #21

8. _____ #22

a. # 3 Short

b. # 3 Long

c. # 7

d. #. 4 Short

e. #. 4 Long

f. # 9

g. Beaver

67

SHORT ANSWERS

Provide a short answer for each question or statement.

1. Explain the difference in a self-retaining retractor and a handheld retractor. Also, give an example of each and the surgical procedure for which you would use the retractor.

   _____

   _____

2. You are the scrub for an exploratory laparotomy, where the surgeon is irrigating the abdomen. What suction tip would you use and why?

   _____

   _____

3. You are the second circulator in the room and the circulator asks you to get an EEA stapler. What type of surgical procedure would you use the stapler for?

   _____

   _____

4. You are scrubbed on an open reduction internal fixation (ORIF) of the ankle, and the surgeon asks for an elevator. What type of elevator would you use and why?

   _____

   _____

5. During a transurethral resection of the prostate (TURP), the surgeon asks for an instrument to relieve a stricture of the urethra. What type of instrument would you give the surgeon?

   _____

   _____

6. You are scrubbed on a thyroidectomy and the surgeon asks for a vessel clip. What type would you give the surgeon and why?

   _____

   _____

7. You are scrubbed on a total knee arthroplasty, and the surgeon asks for an instrument to scrape out a portion of diseased bone. What type of instrument would you give the surgeon?

   _____

   _____

MULTIPLE CHOICE

Choose the correct answer for each question.

1. An example of an angled instrument is a(n):
   a. Schnidt
   b. Mixter
   c. Osteotome
   d. Deaver

2. Which instrument penetrates the tissue rather than just holding it?
   a. Tenaculum
   b. Babcock
   c. Kelly
   d. Lowman

3. Which instrument is used to grasp the fallopian tube or intestinal tissue?
   a. Allen
   b. Babcock
   c. Kocher
   d. Adson

4. All of the following are types of elevators, *except:*
   a. Penfield
   b. Curette
   c. Cobb
   d. Key

5. Which instrument is used to remove bone using a biting action?
   a. Rongeur
   b. Osteotome
   c. Curette
   d. Chisel

6. Which instrument is used to remove excess fluid from the throat?
   a. Poole
   b. Yankauer
   c. Frazier
   d. Joseph

7. Choose the self-retaining retractor that is used during abdominal surgery.
   a. Finochietto
   b. Balfour
   c. Gelpi
   d. Weitlaner

8. Which instrument is used to clamp small blood vessels?
   a. Babcock clamp
   b. Duval lung clamp
   c. Mosquito hemostat
   d. Crile hemostat

9. What classification is a Kocher?
   a. Clamping
   b. Grasping
   c. Retracting
   d. Cutting

10. What classification is a Babcock?
    a. Clamping
    b. Grasping
    c. Retracting
    d. Cutting

11. What classification is a hemostat?
    a. Clamping
    b. Grasping
    c. Retracting
    d. Cutting

12. What classification is a Richardson Eastman?
    a. Clamping
    b. Grasping
    c. Retracting
    d. Cutting

13. Which needle holder has a curved tip?
    a. Baumgartner
    b. Mayo-Hegar
    c. Sarot
    d. Heaney

14. _____ reduces glare but is also prone to staining.
    a. Highly polished or mirror finish
    b. Satin finish
    c. Black chromium
    d. Titanium anodizing

15. _____ instruments resist staining.
    a. Highly polished or mirror finish
    b. Satin finish
    c. Black chromium
    d. Titanium anodizing

16. _____ is a finishing method that imparts color and hardness to the surface of titanium.
    a. Highly polished or mirror
    b. Satin
    c. Black chromium
    d. Titanium anodizing

17. _____ finish is used on laser surgery instruments.
    a. Highly polished or mirror finish
    b. Satin
    c. Black chromium
    d. Titanium anodizing

18. The _____ is a small cup with a sharpened, serrated, or smooth rim at the end of the handle.
    a. Rongeur
    b. Osteotome
    c. Curette
    d. Shears

19. A _____ is used to remodel bone.
    a. Rasp
    b. Curette
    c. Chisel
    d. Osteotome

20. If an instrument has a gold finish on the ring fingers or handle indicates the working tip or edge of the instrument has:
    a. Stainless steel
    b. Tungsten carbide
    c. Chromium
    d. Nickle

21. Supercut scissors have serrations in the cutting edge of the blade. If the surgeon requests a supercut scissor what color handle will you look for on the scissors you have on the back table?
    a. Gold
    b. Anodized
    c. Black
    d. Satin

CASE STUDIES

1. *Briefly describe the following surgical instrument grades and finishes. Be sure to include the materials of which they are made and the purposes for which they are used.*

    a. Surgical-grade instruments

    b. Floor-grade instruments

    c. Bright (or mirror) finish instruments

d. Satin finish instruments

e. Ebony finish instruments

f. Disposable instruments

12 Perioperative Pharmacology

Student's Name _____

KEY TERMS

Write the definition for each term.

1. Adverse reaction: _____.

2. Agonist: _____.

3. Allergy: _____.

4. Antagonist: _____.

5. Antibiotics: _____.

6. Bioavailability: _____.

7. Chemical name: _____.

8. Concentration: _____.

9. Contraindication: _____.

10. Contrast media: _____.

11. Controlled substances: _____.

12. Diluent: _____.

13. Dosage: _____.

14. Dose: _____.

15. Drug: _____.

16. Drug administration: _____.

17. Generation: _____.

18. Generic name: _____.

19. Half-life: _____.

20. Hypersensitivity: _____.

21. Intraosseous: _____.

22. Intrathecal: _____.

23. Parenteral: _____.

24. Peak effect: _____.

72

25. Pharmacodynamics: _____.

26. Pharmacokinetics: _____.

27. Pharmacology: _____.

28. Prescription: _____.

29. Proprietary name: _____.

30. Side effects: _____.

31. Therapeutic window: _____.

32. Topical: _____.

33. Trade name: _____.

34. Transdermal: _____.

35. U.S. Pharmacopeia (USP): _____.

SHORT ANSWERS

Provide a short answer for each question or statement.

1. Drugs used in modern medicine are derived from a number of synthetic and natural sources. Name the sources, and give an example of each.

   _____

   _____

2. The Joint Commission (TJC) requires health care organizations develop policies that agree with state laws regulating who may handle drugs and in what circumstances. What activities must be regulated?

   _____

3. Describe the medication process.

   _____

4. The FDA maintains strict regulatory control on devices and substances used on or in the body, which includes:

   _____

   _____

5. List the four types of allergic reactions, and explain the differences between them.

   a. _____

   b. _____

   c. _____

   d. _____

73

6. Who or what indicates or recommends a route for drug administration to a patient?

_____

_____

7. If you are scrubbed and you are about to label the medication on your table, what information must be on the label?

_____

_____

8. List the 10 elements that have the most influence on drug errors.

a. _____

b. _____

c. _____

d. _____

e. _____

f. _____

g. _____

h. _____

i. _____

j. _____

9. What are the three commonly used staining solutions and what are they used for during the intraoperative period?

a. _____

b. _____

c. _____

10. Name a topical antibiotic commonly used for wound irrigation?

_____

_____

11. What is the difference between a staining agent, a dye, and a contrast medium?

_____

_____

12. What is the difference between colloids and crystalloids? Give an example of each.

   a. Example of a colloid:

   _____

   b. Example of a crystal:

   _____

13. List the seven drug rights and define.

   a. _____

   b. _____

   c. _____

   d. _____

   e. _____

   f. _____

   g. _____

14. List the protocol for receiving and dispensing drugs on the sterile field.

   _____

   _____

15. Using the drug label in Fig. 12.1 in the text, answer these questions:

   a. What is the generic name?

   _____

   b. What is the *proprietary* name?

   _____

   c. What is the dosage form?

   _____

   d. What is the dosage and route of administration?

   _____

   e. What are the contraindications?

   _____

MATCHING

Match each term with the correct definition.

_____ 1. A sterile solution intended to bathe or flush open wounds or body cavities; used topically, never parenterally.

a. Aerosol

b. Capsule

_____ 2. A drug delivery system that often contains an adhesive backing that is applied to an external site on the body.

c. Cement

_____ 3. A solution for the preparation of an iced saline slush, which is administered by irrigation and used to induce regional hypothermia (in conditions such as certain open heart and kidney procedures) by its direct application.

d. Concentrate

e. Cream

_____ 4. A semisolid dosage form that contains a gelling agent to provide stiffness to a solution or colloidal solution or dispersion.

f. Emulsion

g. Film

_____ 5. A product that is packaged under pressure and contains therapeutically active ingredients that are released on activation of an appropriate valve system; it is intended for topical application to the skin as well as local application into the nose (nasal aerosols), mouth (lingual aerosols), or lungs (inhalation aerosols).

h. Gel

i. Graft

j. Implant

_____ 6. An alcoholic or hydroalcoholic solution.

k. Inhalant

_____ 7. An emulsion, semisolid dosage form used for external application to the skin or mucous membranes.

l. Injection

_____ 8. A mixture of dry drugs or chemicals that on addition of suitable vehicles yields a solution.

m. Irrigant

n. Packing

_____ 9. A solid dosage form containing medicinal substances.

o. Patch

_____ 10. A material containing drug intended to be inserted securely or deeply in tissue for growth, slow release, or formation of an organic union.

p. Pellet

_____ 11. A clear homogeneous liquid that contains one or more chemical substances dissolved in a solvent.

q. Pill

_____ 12. A solid oral dosage form consisting of a shell and filling.

r. Plaster

_____ 13. A small piece of flat absorbent material that contains a drug.

s. Powder for solution

_____ 14. Substance intended for external application of consistency to adhere to the skin and attach to a dressing; intended to afford protection and support.

t. Solution

u. Solution for slush

_____ 15. A liquid minutely divided as by a jet or stream of air.

v. Sponge

_____ 16. A liquid preparation of increased strength and reduced volume that is usually diluted before administration.

w. Spray

_____ 17. A small, round, solid dosage form containing a medicinal agent intended for oral administration.

x. Swab

y. Tablet

_____ 18. A porous, interlacing, absorbent material that contains a drug.

z. Tincture

_____ 19. A material usually covered by or impregnated with a drug that is inserted into a body cavity.

_____ 20. A dosage form consisting of at least two immiscible liquids, one of which is dispersed as droplets within the other liquid.

_____ 21. A class of inhalations consisting of a drug or combination of drugs that are carried into the nasal passage, where they exert their effect.

_____ 22. A small sterile solid mass consisting of a highly purified drug intended for implantation in the body.

_____ 23. A sterile preparation intended for parenteral use. Five classes of injections are defined by the USP.

_____ 24. A thin layer or coating.

_____ 25. A slip of skin or other tissue for implantation.

_____ 26. A substance that produces a solid union between two surfaces.

MATCHING

Match the route of administration with the dosage form.

1. _____ Sublingual

2. _____ Intravenous

3. _____ Vaginal

4. _____ Intraosseous (IO)

5. _____ Subcutaneous (SQ)

6. _____ Intradermal (ID)

7. _____ Transdermal

8. _____ Intraperitoneal

9. _____ Ingestion

10. _____ Inhalant

11. _____ Intramuscular (IM)

12. _____ Instillation

13. _____ Rectal

14. _____ Buccal

15. _____ Nasal

16. _____ Intraspinal

a. Parenteral

b. Oral

c. Topical

MATCHING

Match the following blood and blood products.

_____ 1. Concentration of several hemostatic proteins that have been prepared from whole blood.

_____ 2. Essential for blood coagulation containing coagulation factors, RBCs, and white blood cells administered to patients with bleeding disorders.

_____ 3. Extracted from whole blood and contains normal amounts of coagulation factors.

_____ 4. Used in patients with hemophilia who require invasive procedures.

_____ 5. Contains serum and blood cells, plus anticoagulants and preservatives.

_____ 6. Administered to patients who demonstrate repeated hypersensitivity to blood or blood components.

_____ 7. Administered to patients with a history of non-hemolytic febrile transfusion reactions.

_____ 8. Administered to increase the oxygen-carrying capacity of blood.

_____ 9. Obtained from an AO Rh-compatible donor used in treatment of severe neutropenia.

a. Whole blood

b. Granulocytes

c. Packed red blood cells

d. Leukoreduced red blood cells

e. Factor concentrates

f. Washed red blood cells

g. Cryoprecipitate

h. Platelets

i. Fresh frozen plasma

Match the following hemostatic agents and tissue sealants; there may be more than one answer for each item, match all that apply.

1. _____ Fibrant sealant applied to the surface of tissues to bind them together.

2. _____ Collagen absorbable hemostat manufactured from bovine collagen supplied in dry form as powder, sheets, and sponges.

3. _____ Oral anticoagulant using vitamin K antagonist in treatment of venous thromboembolism, pulmonary embolism, and cardiac abnormalities that increase the risk of embolism.

4. _____ Used for the immediate breakdown of systemic blood clots in myocardial infarction, ischemic stroke, and pulmonary embolism.

5. _____ Topical powder applied dry or mixed with isotonic saline for use as a spray, by drop, or soaking sponges.

6. _____ Inhibits blood clot formation but does not dissolve clots.

7. _____ Mesh, granular, or fluff topical mechanical hemostatic agent.

8. _____ Induces blood coagulation.

9. _____ Absorbable dry sponge applied to develop clot formation.

10. _____ Hemostatic material applied to the surface of bleeding bone.

11. _____ Hemostatic material available in mesh, fluff, or powder form.

12. _____ Injectable anticoagulant used in treatment of venous thromboembolism, pulmonary embolism, and cardiac abnormalities that increase the risk of embolism.

a. Coagulant

b. Anticoagulant

c. Thrombolytic drug

d. Warfarin

e. Heparin

f. Floseal

g. Surgiflo

h. Topical thrombin

i. Gelatin

j. Collagen

k. Cellulose

l. Gelfoam

m. Gelfilm

n. Surgifoam

o. Surgical

p. Avitene

q. Bone wax (Ostene)

MATCHING

Match the agents to the conditions they are used for.

1. _____ Used in PACU to prevent or reduce vomiting.

2. _____ Used to treat certain types of cancers.

3. _____ Group of drugs for the body's response in autoimmune disease manifestations.

4. _____ Osmotic diuretic used to reduce cerebral edema and intraocular pressure.

5. _____ Used to treat bacterial infections.

6. _____ Used to manage insulin.

7. _____ Used to stimulate production of urine by the kidneys.

8. _____ Used to treat superficial and systemic fungal infections.

9. _____ Used to augment contractions during labor.

10. _____ Used in the treatment of asthma and during anesthesia emergencies such as anaphylactic shock.

11. _____ Used to control airway secretions and to regulate heart rate in selected patients.

a. Corticosteroid

b. Antidiabetic

c. Oxytocin

d. Antibiotic

e. Antifungal

f. Antineoplastic

g. Anticholinergics

h. Adrenergic

i. Diuretic

j. Mannitol

k. Antiemetic

MATCHING

Match the anesthetic agents to their function.

_____ 1. Natural or synthetic opiates used for moderate to severe pain control.

_____ 2. Inhalation anesthetic safely used for both adults and pediatric patients, with a rapid emergence causing it to be useful for outpatient surgery.

_____ 3. Reduces anxiety and provides muscle relaxation.

_____ 4. Used in conjunction with general anesthesia to paralyze skeletal muscles, as an essential component to anesthesia.

_____ 5. Commonly used for the induction of anesthesia, additionally for treatment of seizure disorders.

_____ 6. Used for induction and maintenance used in low doses on short procedures for short surgical procedures that do not require unconsciousness.

_____ 7. Short rapid-acting dissociative anesthesia that can cause delirium in adults.

_____ 8. Widely used inhalation anesthetic with systemic effects superior to other inhalation agents.

_____ 9. The most common intravenous sedative used for induction and maintenance of general anesthesia.

_____ 10. Colorless, odorless inhalation anesthetic delivered in a gaseous form.

_____ 11. Inhalation anesthetic ideal for outpatient surgery providing rapid emergence used on adults but not used with pediatric patients due to a high incidence of bronchospasm and laryngospasm.

a. Benzodiazepine

b. Barbiturate

c. Ketamine

d. Propofol

e. Narcotic

f. Neuromuscular blocking agent

g. Nitrous oxide

h. Isoflurane

i. Sevoflurane

j. Desflurane

k. Enflurane (Ethrane)

80

MULTIPLE CHOICE

1. Which of the following osmotic diuretics is used to reduce intraocular pressure and cerebral edema?
   a. Rantidine
   b. Mannitol
   c. Prednisol
   d. Ergometrine

2. Shich of the following medications can be administered intravenously?
   a. Gelfoam
   b. Thrombin
   c. Ostene
   d. Heparin

3. Using the federal drug schedules of controlled substances, which schedule of drug has a high potential for abuse and has an accepted medical use with restrictions in the United States in which the abuse can lead to severe psychological of physical dependence?
   a. Schedule I
   b. Schedule II
   c. Schedule III
   d. Schedule IV

4. Drugs used to reduce the bodys immune response are _____.
   a. Diuretics
   b. Anticholinergics
   c. Antiinfective
   d. Corticosteroids

5. Which type of drugs administered in the PACU to prevent or reduce nausea and vomiting postoperatively?
   a. Antiemetic agent
   b. Histamine receptor
   c. Anticholinergic
   d. Adrenegic

CASE STUDY

Read the following case study and answer the questions at the end of the case study.

1. You are assigned to relieve on a lunch break in room 2. The surgical technologist you are relieving reports off to you counts and medications in the field. You notice none of the medications, syringes, or irrigation solutions are labeled. What should you do?

Student's Name _____

KEY TERMS

Write the definition for each term.

1. Airway: _____

2. Amnesia: _____

3. Analgesia: _____

4. Anesthesia: _____

5. Anesthesia care provider (ACP)(AP): _____

6. Anesthesia machine: _____

7. Anesthesia technician: _____

8. Anesthesiologist: _____

9. Anesthetic: _____

10. Amnesia: _____

11. Anxiolytic: _____

12. Apnea: _____

13. Auscultation: _____

14. Aspiration: _____

15. Bier block: _____

16. Breathing bag: _____

17. Bronchospasm: _____

18. Central nervous system depression: _____

19. Coma: _____

20. Consciousness: _____

21. Delirium: _____

22. Discharge against medical advice: _____

23. Emergence: _____

24. Endotracheal tube: _____

25. Esmarch bandage: _____

26. Extubation: _____

27. Gas scavenging: _____

28. General anesthesia: _____

29. Glasgow coma scale: _____

30. Handover: _____

31. Homeostasis: _____

32. Hypothermia: _____

33. Induction: _____

34. Intraoperative awareness (IOA): _____

35. Intravascular volume: _____

36. Intubation: _____

37. Laryngeal mask airway (LMA): _____

38. Laryngoscope: _____

39. Laryngospasm: _____

40. Malignant hyperthermia (MH): _____

41. Moderate sedation: _____

42. Monitored anesthesia care (MAC): _____

43. Nasopharyngeal airway: _____

44. Neuromuscular blocking agent: _____

45. Oropharyngeal airway (OPA): _____

46. Perfusion: _____

47. Physiological monitoring: _____

48. Pneumatic tourniquet: _____

49. Postanesthesia care unit (PACU): _____

50. Preoperative medication: _____

51. Protective reflexes: _____

52. Pulmonary embolism (PE): _____

53. Pulse oximeter: _____

54. Regional block: _____

55. Sedation: _____

56. Sedative: _____

57. Sensation: _____

58. Topical anesthesia: _____

59. Unconsciousness: _____

LABELING

Label the laryngeal mask.

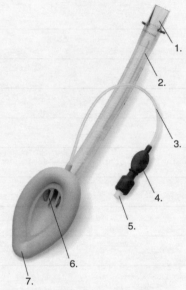

Courtesy LMA North America.

1. _____

2. _____

3. _____

4. _____

5. _____

6. _____

7. _____

SHORT ANSWERS

Provide a short answer for each question or statement.

1. Anesthesia means "without sensation." What is the goal of surgical anesthesia?

_____

_____

2. List the primary goal of the ACP.

_____

3. What seven things help the surgeon, the ACP, and the patient decide which type of anesthetic will be best for the individual during the procedure?

a. _____

b. _____

c. _____

d. _____

e. _____

f. _____

g. _____

4. Hospitals and other surgical facilities have individual check-in protocols. Which specific details are always verified?

a. _____

a. _____

c. _____

d. _____

e. _____

f. _____

g. _____

h. _____

i. _____

5. What are the four phases/stages of anesthesia?

a. _____

b. _____

c. _____

d. _____

MATCHING

Match each term with the correct definition.

_____ 1. Diminished mental, sensory, and physical capacity. It is another way of expressing sedation.

_____ 2. The loss of recall (memory) of events.

_____ 3. Loss of pain sensation. Specialized nerves transmit signals from the source of pain to the brain. Particular drugs interrupt these pain nerve pathways.

_____ 4. The awareness of stimuli, including hearing, sight, smell, taste, touch, temperature (heat and cold), pressure, and pain.

_____ 5. The deepest state of unconsciousness, in which most brain activity ceases.

_____ 6. A state of awareness in which a person is able to *sense the environment and respond to it.*

_____ 7. Severe depression of the central nervous system (CNS) resulting in the *inability to respond to external stimuli.* Deep unconsciousness, such as that achieved during general anesthesia, results in the absence of protective mechanisms, such as swallowing, coughing, blinking, and shivering.

_____ 8. A *state of consciousness* described along a continuum. At one end, a person is fully aware of the surroundings and able to respond to stimuli. At the other end is unconsciousness, in which the patient is not aware of the environment and cannot respond to external stimuli including those that are noxious (e.g., pain, cold, heat).

a. Sensation

b. Analgesia

c. Consciousness

d. Sedation

e. Central nervous system depression

f. Unconsciousness

g. Coma

h. Amnesia

MATCHING

Match each parameter measured with the physiological monitoring device.

Parameters measured:

_____ 1. Core body temperature

_____ 2. Rapid administration of fluids and bloods

_____ 3. Myocardial ischemia

_____ 4. Detects air embolism

_____ 5. Assess valve function

_____ 6. Assessment of cardiac preload

_____ 7. Auscultation of breathing and heart sounds

_____ 8. Measures central venous pressure

_____ 9. Ventilator disconnection during general anesthesia

_____ 10. Blood oxygen saturation

_____ 11. Heart rate

_____ 12. Measurement of arterial blood pressure

_____ 13. Evaluates myocardium

_____ 14. Cardiac preload

_____ 15. Heart rate

_____ 16. Heart rhythm

_____ 17. Adequacy of ventilation

_____ 18. Delivered oxygen concentration

_____ 19. Gross indication of renal perfusion and intravascular volume

_____ 20. Assessment of descending aortic flow

_____ 21. Monitor airway pressure

_____ 22. Blood pressure

_____ 23. Obtain samples of arterial blood for analysis

_____ 24. Detection of air embolism

_____ 25. Airway pressure

_____ 26. Assess intravascular volume

_____ 27. Cardiac output

_____ 28. Drug administration

a. Pulse oximetry

b. Automatic blood pressure cuff

c. Electrocardiography

d. Capnography

e. Oxygen analyzer

f. Ventilator pressure monitor

g. Temperature-monitoring probe (Foley type)

h. Urine output using Foley catheter

i. Central venous catheter

j. Arterial catheter

k. Precordial doppler

l. Transesophageal cchocardiography

m. Esophageal doppler

n. Transpulmonary indicator dilution

o. Esophageal and precordial stethoscope

Chapter **13** **Anesthesia, Physiological Monitoring, and Post Anesthesia Recovery**

MATCHING

Match the type of regional anesthesia to method of anesthesia delivery

_____ 1. Intravenous block where blood is temporarily displaced from a limb and replaced by a local anesthetic with use of a pneumatic tourniquet.

_____ 2. Injection of an anesthetic into superficial tissues to produce a small area of anesthesia.

_____ 3. Anesthesia applied on skin, mucous membranes, and superficial eye tissues.

_____ 4. Anesthesia agent injected into tissue to anesthetize a group of fine superficial nerves in a small area.

_____ 5. Anesthesia injected into the epidural space often used for OB GYN.

_____ 6. Injection of anesthesia into the subarachnoid space.

a. Topical anesthesia

b. Local infiltration

c. Nerve block

d. Bier block

e. Spinal anesthesia

f. Epidural

MULTIPLE CHOICE

Choose the most correct answer to complete the question or statement.

1. _____ is an invasive airway that extends from the mouth to the trachea.
   a. OPA (Oropharyngeal airway)
   b. LMA (Laryngeal mask airway)
   c. NPA (Nasopharyngeal airway)
   d. ET tube (Endotracheal tube)

2. _____ provides passage between the nostril and the nasopharynx.
   a. OPA (Oropharyngeal airway)
   b. LMA (Laryngeal mask airway)
   c. NPA (Nasopharyngeal airway)
   d. ET tube (Endotracheal tube)

3. _____ is inserted over the tongue to prevent the tongue or epiglottis from falling back against the pharynx.
   a. OPA (Oropharyngeal airway)
   b. LMA (Laryngeal mask airway)
   c. NPA (Nasopharyngeal airway)
   d. ET tube (Endotracheal tube)

4. _____ is inserted without the aid of a laryngoscope and fits snugly over the larynx.
   a. OPA (Oropharyngeal airway)
   b. LMA (Laryngeal mask airway)
   c. NPA (Nasopharyngeal airway)
   d. ET tube (Endotracheal tube)

5. The _____ phase involves continuation of the anesthetic agent.
   a. Induction
   b. Maintenance
   c. Emergence
   d. Recovery

6. Post-anesthesia care is provided in the _____ phase.
   a. Induction
   b. Maintenance
   c. Emergence
   d. Recovery

7. During the _____ phase, general anesthesia begins with the administration of the drug ending with loss of consciousness.
   a. Induction
   b. Maintenance
   c. Emergence
   d. Recovery

8. The _____ phase is the withdrawing of the anesthetic.
   a. Induction
   b. Maintenance
   c. Emergence
   d. Recovery

9. During _____ the patient is relaxed, and protective reflexes are lost.
   a. Stage 1
   b. Stage 2
   c. Stage 3
   d. Stage 4

10. _____ begins with the administration of induction drugs and ends with loss of consciousness.
    a. Stage 1
    b. Stage 2
    c. Stage 3
    d. Stage 4

11. During what stage can anesthesia overdose resulting in severe respiratory and circulatory collapse occur?
    a. Stage 1
    b. Stage 2
    c. Stage 3
    d. Stage 4

12. During _____, delirium ensues, marked by unconsciousness and exaggerated reflexes.
    a. Stage 1
    b. Stage 2
    c. Stage 3
    d. Stage 4

13. _____ is induced with the drug ketamine.
    a. Dissociative anesthesia
    b. Regional anesthesia
    c. Conscious sedation
    d. Nonreceptive sedation

14. _____ provides reversible loss of sensation in a specific area of the body without affecting consciousness.
    a. Dissociative anesthesia
    b. Regional anesthesia
    c. Conscious sedation
    d. Nonreceptive sedation

15. MAC stands for:
    a. Monitored anesthesia consciousness
    b. Monitored anesthetic care
    c. Monitored anesthesia care
    d. None of the above

16. A _____ anesthetic is an injection into superficial tissue to produce a small area of anesthesia.
    a. Topical
    b. Local
    c. Spinal
    d. Nerve

17. A _____ anesthetic provides anesthesia to a specific area of the body supplied by a major nerve or nerve plexus.
    a. Topical
    b. Local
    c. Spinal
    d. Nerve

18. A _____ anesthetic is used on mucous membranes and on superficial eye tissue during ophthalmic surgery.
    a. Topical
    b. Local
    c. Spinal
    d. Nerve

19. A(n) _____ is injection of anesthetic into the intrathecal space.
    a. Intravenous block
    b. Nerve block
    c. Epidural
    d. Spinal block

20. A _____ is a also known as Bier block.
    a. Intravenous block
    b. Nerve
    c. Epidural
    d. Spinal

21. A _____ is produced when the anesthetic agent is injected into the epidural space.
    a. Intravenous block
    b. Nerve block
    c. Epidural
    d. Spinal block

22. When the body is in a balanced physiological state, it is in:
    a. Hemostasis
    b. Balanced anesthesia
    c. Homeostasis
    d. Topical anesthesia

23. Electrocardiography (ECG) measures the:
    a. Heart rate per minute
    b. Electrical activity of the brain
    c. Electrical activity of the heart
    d. Respiratory rate per minute

24. Which of the following would *not* be needed for a Bier block procedure?
    a. Enflurane
    b. Esmarch bandage
    c. IV
    d. Pneumatic tourniquet

25. Type of shock caused by severe bacterial infection resulting in hypovolemia is called:
    a. Hypovolemic
    b. Cardiogenic
    c. Anaphylaxis
    d. Septic

26. Type of shock is the depletion of the total intravascular volume caused by redistribution of body fluids from trauma or burn, or external fluid loss from vomiting, diarrhea, polyuria, or blood lost is called:
    a. Hypovolemic
    b. Cardiogenic
    c. Anaphylaxis
    d. Septic

27. Rare physiological response to all volatile anesthetic agents and succinylcholine, symptoms including high core temperature, tachycardia, tachypnea, and increased muscle rigidity is called:
    a. Hemorrhage
    b. Shock
    c. Malignant hyperthermia
    d. Laryngospasm

28. Dantrolene (Dantrium) is an emergency drug used to treat:
    a. Cardiopulmonary arrest
    b. Malignant hyperthermia
    c. Septic shock
    d. Hypovolemic shock

29. _____ complications can be managed by an anelgesic.
    a. Respiratory
    b. Pain
    c. Cardiovascular
    d. Metabolic

30. The patient history includes all of the following, *except*:
    a. Age
    b. Allergies
    c. Current medications
    d. Future pathology

31. After receiving the handover, the PACU nurse performs a patient:
    a. Head-to-toe assessment
    b. Pain assessment
    c. Social assessment
    d. Wound assessment

32. Bowel sounds are assessed by:
    a. Observation
    b. Palpation
    c. X-ray
    d. Auscultation

33. Assessment for dehydration includes:
    a. Cardiac dysrhythmia
    b. Alteration in consciousness
    c. Physical signs and symptoms
    d. Blood tests

34. Patients are discharged from the PACU only when they:
    a. Meet discharge criteria
    b. Meet the respiratory standards
    c. Achieve PACU standards
    d. Become normotensive

35. Your male surgical patient is about to be discharged from PACU. Which of the following does *not* meet the criteria for discharge?
    a. The patient arranged for transportation before being admitted for the procedure.
    b. The PACU has called a cab to deliver the patient to his apartment.
    c. The patient has asked his friend to assist him to his home.
    d. The patient's mother has arrived to drive him home and stay with him for the day.

36. It is the responsibility of _____ to educate the patient before the individual is discharged from the hospital to go home.
    a. The surgical technologist
    b. The surgeon
    c. The anesthesia care provider
    d. Nursing personnel trained in discharge planning

CASE STUDY

1. *You are about to scrub in on a case and the anesthesia care provider informs you and the circulator that the patient has a family member who has experienced malignant hyperthermia in the past.*

   a. What should you do prior to surgery in preparation for the case?

b. What items are available on the malignant hyperthermia cart?

c. The procedure has begun and the ACP alerts the team the patient is exhibiting an extremely high core temperature, tachycardia, tachypnea and increased muscle rigidity. What should you do?

14 Death and Dying

Student's Name _____

KEY TERMS

Write the definition for each term.

1. Advance health care directive: _____

2. Coroner's case: _____

3. Cultural competence: _____

4. Determination of death: _____

5. DNAR: _____

6. DNR: _____

7. End of life: _____

8. Heart beating cadaver: _____

9. Kübler-Ross, Elisabeth: _____

10. Living will: _____

11. Non–heart beating cadaver: _____

12. Postmortem care: _____

13. Required request law: _____

14. Rigor mortis: _____

SHORT ANSWER

Provide a short answer for each question or statement.

1. From a medical point of view, the *end of life* is:

_____

_____

2. The term *brain* dead refers to:

_____

_____

3. _____ is the right of every individual to make decisions about how he or she lives and dies.

4. _____ issues arise when decisions about end-of-life care fall to the family when the patient is unable to communicate his or her wishes.

5. _____ or _____ expresses the patient decision to decline lifesaving efforts.

6. _____ care is the medical and supportive care provided to the dying patient.

7. Describe briefly the difference between a living will and a DNR order.

_____

_____

8. The surgical technologist should refrain from providing information to family or friends about _____ of the patient.

MATCHING

Match the term with the description.

1. _____ It may occur during the dying process, but treated clinically. a. Denial

2. _____ A natural first response, a defense mechanism. b. Bargaining

3. _____ The idea that death is no longer a source of psychological conflict. c. Anger

4. _____ Refusing nutrition or treatment. d. Acceptance

5. _____ "I just want to experience one pain-free day with my family." e. Depression

MULTIPLE CHOICE

Choose the most correct answer to complete the question or statement.

1. Which of the following is a famous physiatrist who constructed the death and dying model that is most frequently recognized today?
   a. Maslow
   b. Freud
   c. Piaget
   d. Elisabeth Kübler-Ross

2. During the dying process, _____ is a defense mechanism that forestalls the full impact of the fact of death until the mind is ready to accept it.
   a. Denial
   b. Acceptance
   c. Bargaining
   d. Anger

3. A dying patient may express anger to:
   a. Gain control over the environment
   b. Get even with the physician
   c. Pass through the stages of dying even if the person is not angry
   d. Keep from becoming depressed

4. It is the responsibility of the _____ to convey information about the patient's medical condition to the family and/or friends.
   a. Operating room scheduler or secretary
   b. Surgeon only
   c. Physician and nurses
   d. Operating room staff

5. The order to _____ is made official by signing a DNR order, which is charted in the patient's medical record.
   a. Not resuscitate
   b. Call the doctor
   c. Add additional medications
   d. Sign a surgical consent form

6. Examples of palliative care include all of the following, *except*:
   a. Debulking of a tumor
   b. X-ray films
   c. Debridement of a pressure wound
   d. Insertion of a gastric feeding tube

93

7. If there is a sudden death in the operating room, it is appropriate for the technologist only to:
   a. Provide details about the cause of death
   b. Provide details about what occurred in the operating room
   c. Offer an acknowledgment of loss
   d. Discuss the laboratory test values

8. For surgical technologists to recognize and acknowledge the fact of death and what this means to the patient in that moment and time, they should:
   a. Focus on what the patient is experiencing in the operating room or holding area
   b. Observe facial expressions and gestures
   c. Be alert to any changes in mood or signs of anxiety and fear related to death and isolation
   d. All of the above

9. Medical interventions for a dying patient include all of the following, *except:*
   a. Respiratory support (artificial respiration)
   b. Intravenous feeding
   c. Dialysis
   d. Pain medications

10. The _____ of death is considered by some to be too constricting and does not allow for individualism in the experience of death.
    a. Stage theory
    b. End-of-life theory
    c. Spiritual theory
    d. Psychological theory
    e. Examination

11. _____ is the right of every individual to make decisions about how he or she lives and dies.
    a. DNR
    b. Advance directive
    c. Self-determination
    d. Living will

12. A _____ specifies the exact nature of palliative care that a patient accepts.
    a. Living will
    b. Advance directive
    c. DNR
    d. Assisted suicide

13. When no verifiable permission has been granted for organ donation by the patient, the _____ may act as a surrogate for the patient.
    a. Surgeon
    b. Family
    c. Chaplain
    d. Nurses

14. In the operating room, death is a(n) _____ event.
    a. Rare
    b. Occasional
    c. Weekly
    d. Daily

15. For a coroner's case, all of the following are mandatory for an autopsy, *except:*
    a. Death of an incarcerated individual
    b. Unwitnessed death
    c. Death from a diagnosed terminal illness in which the patient was being treated for
    d. Suicide

16. Donors are registered in different _____ of the country and the data are exchanged with recovery organizations.
    a. Parts
    b. States
    c. Regions
    d. Counties

17. Reactions and coping skills available to health care professionals are influenced by the following factors, *except:*
    a. Lack of support
    b. The health care professional's beliefs and values
    c. Previous experience with death
    d. Emotional well-being

18. A _____ cadaver is maintained on cardiopulmonary support to provide tissue perfusion.
    a. Non-heart-beating
    b. Heart-beating

19. The cornea, bone and skin can be harvested from a _____ cadaver.
    a. Non–heart-beating
    b. Heart-beating

20. Organ and tissue donation arises as a(n) _____ issue when the patient has not left a clear directive before death.
    a. Moral
    b. Ethical

21. _____ prepares the body for viewing by the family and assists in further handling procedures carried out by the morgue and mortuary.
    a. Rigor mortis
    b. Operating room
    c. Postmortem care
    d. All the above

22. The process of recovery is administered through:
    a. Donors
    b. Tissue banks
    c. Recipients
    d. Organized recovery
    e. All the above

CASE STUDIES

1. *Read the following case study and answer the questions based on your knowledge of death and dying.*

   You are called in for an exploratory laparotomy. Upon arrival to the hospital, you learn your patient has a ruptured aneurysm. You prepare the operating room and scrub, then notice the patient is brought in and is not breathing. The surgeon makes the incision and the abdomen is filled with blood and your patient crashes. After a very brief silence, you patient dies on the table.

   a. What is your role as a surgical technologist at this point?

   b. The patient's family wants to see their family member. Who stays with the family while they say goodbye?

   c. What is the ethical thing to do with this patient?

   d. Do you remove all the cords, clean the patient up before the family visit? Why?

15 Energy Sources in Surgery

Student's Name _____

KEY TERMS

Write the definition for each term.

1. Ablation: _____

2. Active electrode: _____

3. Argon: _____

4. Bipolar circuit: _____

5. Capacitive coupling: _____

6. Carbon dioxide: _____

7. Cavitron ultrasonic surgical aspirator (CUSA): _____

8. Coagulum: _____

9. Cryoablation: _____

10. Cryosurgery: _____

11. Cutting mode: _____

12. Direct coupling: _____

13. Dispersive electrode: _____

14. Electrosurgery: _____

15. Electrosurgical unit (ESU): _____

16. Electrosurgical vessel sealing: _____

17. Eschar: _____

18. Excimer: _____

19. Fulguration: _____

20. Holmium: YAG: _____

21. Impedance: _____

22. Implanted electronic device (IED): _____

23. Insulate: _____

24. Laser: _____

25. Laser classifications: _____

26. Laser head: _____

27. Laser medium: _____

28. Monopolar circuit: _____

29. Nonconductive: _____

30. Optical resonant cavity: _____

31. Patient return electrode (PRE): _____

32. Phacoemulsification: _____

33. Potassium-titanyl-phosphate (KTP): _____

34. Pulsed wave lasers: _____

35. Q-switched lasers: _____

36. Radiant exposure: _____

37. Radiofrequency: _____

38. Return electrode monitoring (REM): _____

39. Selective absorption: _____

40. Smoke plume: _____

41. Ultrasonic energy: _____

LABELING

Name the bovie tip and description of use.

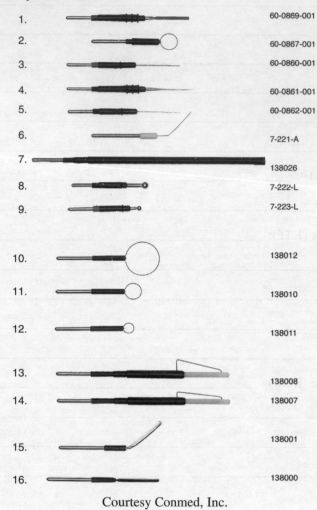

1.   60-0869-001

2.   60-0867-001

3.   60-0860-001

4.   60-0861-001

5.   60-0862-001

6.   7-221-A

7.   138026

8.   7-222-L

9.   7-223-L

10.   138012

11.   138010

12.   138011

13.   138008

14.   138007

15.   138001

16.   138000

Courtesy Conmed, Inc.

1. _____

2. _____

3. _____

4. _____

5. _____

6. _____

7. _____

8. _____

9. _____

10. _____

11. _____

12. _____

13. _____

14. _____

15. _____

16. _____

SHORT ANSWERS

Provide a short answer for each question or statement.

1. Which variables cause tissue to react to electrosurgery?

_____

_____

2. Describe the difference between electrosurgery and ultrasonic energy.

_____

_____

3. What is the difference between monopolar and bipolar delivery of ESU?

_____

_____

4. What is capacitive coupling and why would it occur in endoscopic procedures more often than in open procedures?

_____

_____

5. How do lasers work?

_____

_____

6. How are lasers classified?

_____

_____

7. Lasers are grouped into two categories according to the duration of the output waves. What are the two groups?

a. _____

b. _____

MATCHING

Match each laser classification with the correct definition.

1. _____ Laser printers.

2. _____ Can cause severe eye injury when viewed directly or by reflection. These lasers do not cause injury when the laser beam is diffused and do not normally present a fire hazard.

3. _____ Can cause permanent eye damage if viewed directly or if viewed indirectly by reflection, may also ignite materials and cause skin burns. Most surgical lasers are in this category.

4. _____ Laser pointers and bar code scanners.

5. _____ Normally does not cause eye injury if viewed momentarily but presents a hazard if viewed with collecting optics (e.g., fiberoptic cable, magnification loupe, or microscope.)

a. Class 4

b. Class 3b

c. Class 3a

d. Class 2

e. Class 1

MATCHING

Match the laser with the correct description.

1. _____ Invisible to the human eye, and the beam has a high affinity for water, and functions at a superficial depth.

2. _____ Has a high affinity for tissue protein but little for water. Of all the laser types, has the greatest ability to coagulate blood vessels.

3. _____ A laser that offers two wavelengths, which allows two separate sets of laser characteristics to be selected at any time.

4. _____ This laser beam is outside the visible light range, penetrates all types of tissue, and is extremely versatile, able to cut, shave, contour, ablate, and coagulate tissue.

5. _____ This laser produces a cool beam by stripping electrons from the atoms of the medium in the chambers stimulating short bursts of laser light delivered to target tissue through fiberoptic bundles.

6. _____ Solid lasing material used to remove superficial skin defects and tattoos.

7. _____ A visible blue-green beam that is absorbed by red-brown pigmented tissue, such as hemoglobin.

8. _____ This pulsed dye laser beam is formed when fluorescent liquid or other dyes are exposed to argon laser light.

a. Argon gas laser

b. Carbon dioxide laser

c. Holmium:YAG laser

d. Nd:YAG laser

e. KTP laser

f. Excimer laser

g. Tunable dye laser

h. Ruby and alexandrite

MULTIPLE CHOICE

Choose the most correct answer to complete the question or statement.

1. Resistance to the flow of electricity:
   a. Impedance
   b. Frequency
   c. Circuit
   d. Current

2. The cutting mode causes tissue burning with the loss of water content is:
   a. Blended mode
   b. Cryoablation
   c. Desiccation
   d. Electrosurgical waveforms

3. The _____ provides radio frequency powers and controls for all types of ESU.
   a. Generator
   b. Duty cycle
   c. Desiccation
   d. Electrosurgical waveforms

4. Electrosurgical vessel sealing uses high-frequency, bipolar electrosurgery, low voltage, and physical pressure to create a weld in tissue. All of the follow are true statements, *except:*
   a. The vessel-sealing system is used during resection procedures that traditionally do not require clamping, suturing, and cutting.
   b. Electrosurgical vessel sealing uses a microprocessor that controls and programs the system.
   c. The vessel sealing system provides tissue impedance monitoring.
   d. Electrosurgical vessel sealing system has an alarm that automatically stops the current when the tissue seal is achieved.

5. _____ is a specific burn hazard of monopolar endoscopic surgery, occurring when current passes unintentionally through instrument insulation.
   a. Direct coupling
   b. Capacitive coupling

6. The safety system used in ESU monitoring impedance in the electrode stopping the current if is too high:
   a. PAE
   b. REM

7. _____ is the flow of electricity from one conductive substance to another.
   a. Direct coupling
   b. Capacitive coupling

8. The active electrode is the actual contact point at the tissue and is contained at the:
   a. Tip of the electrosurgical unit (ESU) handpiece or "pencil"
   b. Grounding plate
   c. Generator's plug in
   d. Foot pedal

9. The function of the _____ is to capture electrical current from the active electrode and transmit it back to the power unit.
   a. Bipolar circuit
   b. Bayonet
   c. Return electrode
   d. Pencil type of handpiece

10. In the _____ mode, the electrode is held above the tissue, without contact, and the air between the electrode and tissue acts as a conductor, allowing the high-voltage current to flow between the tissue and the electrode.
    a. Blended
    b. Cutting
    c. Desiccation
    d. Microbipolar cutting

11. Procedure in which a probe is inserted into a tumor or tissue mass. High-pressure argon gas is injected into the probe causing the tissues to freeze destroying the tissue.
    a. Ultrasound
    b. Phacoemulsification
    c. Cryoablation
    d. Laser

12. When laser light is directed at a surface, which of the following would *not* occur?
    a. Absorption
    b. Coagulation
    c. Reflection
    d. Scattering

13. _____ is the use of an extremely cold probe or substance to destroy tissue.
    a. Ultrasound
    b. Phacoemulsification
    c. Cryoablation
    d. Cryosurgery

14. _____ is created when electricity is transformed into mechanical energy generated by high-frequency vibrations and the focus on friction.
    a. Ultrasound
    b. Phacoemulsification
    c. Cryoablation
    d. Ultrasonic energy

15. _____ is performed by inserting a series of needle probes directly into the tumor under direct fluoroscopic imaging.
    a. Ultrasound
    b. Phacoemulsification
    c. Ablation
    d. Cryosurgery

16. Placement of the patient return electrode is extremely important when placing the grounding pad. Which of the following is incorrect related to placement of the pad?
    a. Place on a large muscle
    b. Place over a bony prominence
    c. Have complete contact with the skin surface
    d. Inspect the patients skin before applying the grounding pad

101

17. Where should the ESU pencil placed during surgery?
    a. On top of the patient
    b. On top of the drapes
    c. Tucked under the neck of the patient
    d. In a nonconductive safety holder

18. Forcep style ESU that the circuit flows from the generator through the cable to the tips of the forcep.
    a. Monopolar
    b. Bipolar
    c. Cryosurgery
    d. Ultrasound

19. Protective eyewear for laser procedures must:
    a. Have a clear lens
    b. Bear an inscription on the lens detailing the optical density and label of the specific laser type
    c. Have an opening on the sides of the eyes
    d. Have a clear amber lens

20. When a smoke evacuator is used to suction the smoke plume from the surgical site the tip of the nozzle must be within _____ of the site to be effective.
    a. 2 inches
    b. 4 inches
    c. 6 inches
    d. 1 foot

21. Both laser and ESU plumes contain:
    a. Dead and living cells
    b. Hydrogen cyanide
    c. Formaldehyde and acrolein
    d. Biological particles, such as cancer cells
    c. All of the above

CASE STUDIES

1. Your patient is coming to surgery today, and your surgeon would like to use the laser in the procedure. What safety precautions will the operating room team have to understand and undertake before the laser is used for the patient's procedure?

16 Moving, Handling, and Positioning the Surgical Patient

Student's Name _____

KEY TERMS

Write the definition for each term.

1. Abduction: _____

2. Compression injury: _____

3. Dependent area of the body: _____

4. Embolism: _____

5. Fowler position _____

6. Gurney: _____

7. Hyperextension: _____

8. Hyperflexion: _____

9. Ischemia: _____

10. Kraske position: _____

11. Lateral transfer: _____

12. Lateral position: _____

13. Lithotomy position: _____

14. Range of motion: _____

15. Reverse Trendelenburg: _____

16. Roller board: _____

17. Shearing injury: _____

18. Transfer board: _____

19. Trendelenburg position: _____

LABELING

Label the operating room table in the following figure.

1. _____

2. _____

3. _____

4. _____

5. _____

6. _____

7. _____

8. _____

9. _____

10. _____

11. _____

Modified from Martin JT, Warner MA: *Positioning in anesthesia and surgery*, ed 3, Philadelphia, 1997, WB Saunders.

SHORT ANSWERS

Provide a short answer for each question or statement.

1. What type of activity would or could cause a shearing injury?

_____

_____

2. Health care workers are at risk for skeletal injury while moving and transferring patients. List guidelines for preventing injuries to themselves when moving and handling patients.

_____

_____

3. Accident and injury to patients can be reduced when individuals take responsibility for the possible risks. List causes of injury to the patient when moving and handling the patient during transport and transfer.

_____

_____

_____

4. What are the guidelines that all health care workers should use to identify and validate the patient's identity?

_____

_____

_____

5. List the steps used to perform the log roll and assisted lateral transfer for the patient from a gurney to the operating room table.

_____

_____

MATCHING

Match each term with the correct definition. Some terms may be used more than once.

1. _____ Position in which the patient's head is tilted down.

2. _____ Position in which the patient is lying on the back.

3. _____ Sitting position.

4. _____ Position in which the patient's feet are tilted down.

5. _____ Position in which the patient is lying with the front of the body (the abdomen) on the operating room table.

6. _____ Position used for gynecological, urology, and some rectal procedures.

7. _____ Position used for head, neck, eye, ear, breast, abdominal, and vascular procedures.

8. _____ A type of prone position in which the patient's hips are flexed.

9. _____ Sitting position used for cranial, facial, and reconstructive breast procedures.

10. _____ Side-lying position.

11. _____ Position used for access to the perianal region, buttocks, posterior spine, and posterior lower legs.

12. _____ Position used for anorectal procedures.

13. _____ Position used to provide exposure to the lateral flank and lateral thorax.

14. _____ Position to access the lower abdominal and pelvic organs.

15. _____ Position used for procedures of the upper abdomen and neck.

a. Reverse Trendelenburg position

b. Prone position

c. Lithotomy position

d. Trendelenburg position

e. Supine position

f. Jackknife (Kraske) position

g. Lateral position

h. Fowler position

i. Modified Fowler

j. Lateral decubitis

MATCHING

Match the potential sources of injury with the correct term.

1. _____ Flexion of a joint beyond its normal anatomical range.

2. _____ Tissue injury caused by continuous pressure over an area.

3. _____ Loss of skin and deep tissue related to continuous pressure over an area of the body.

4. _____ Loss of blood supply to a body part either by compression or blockage of the blood vessels, can cause tissue death from lack of oxygen to the tissue.

5. _____ Skin inflammation that can occur when a patient is pulled over a high friction of surface such as a bed sheet or blanker.

6. _____ Extension of a joint beyond its normal anatomical range.

a. Decubitus ulcer

b. Shearing injury

c. Compression injury

d. Hyperextension

e. Hyperflexion

f. Ischemia

MULTIPLE CHOICE

Choose the most correct answer to complete the question or statement.

1. Which of the following terms means movement of a joint or body part away from the body?
   a. Abduction
   b. Adduction
   c. Hyperextension
   d. Ischemia

2. Health care workers are at high risk for injury while caring for, moving, and transferring patients because:
   a. They do not use proper body mechanics when moving a patient.
   b. The tasks are unpredictable.
   c. A sudden shift of the patient's weight may put the worker off balance.
   d. All of the above.

3. Transport and transfer injuries occur more often when:
   a. There is sufficient help.
   b. Personnel assisting in the transfer or transport have a plan.
   c. Personnel are rushed.
   d. The patient is cooperative.

4. Which of the following statements is true regarding patient transfers?
   a. One person should be in charge of the move and guide the others.
   b. It is best to make a plan as you move the patient so that the move is individualized.
   c. The patient's right to modesty is forfeited at admission.
   d. It is best to move the patient without blankets so that the patient does not get tangled up in them.

5. The most important part of transporting patients is:
   a. Proper identification before you transport them
   b. Proper positioning on the cart
   c. Keeping the patient warm while in the hallways
   d. Greeting the patient in a friendly manner and introducing yourself

6. The first step in transferring a mobile patient to a stretcher is to:
   a. Lower the bed rails and align the patient's bed and the stretcher
   b. Make sure the locks are engaged on both the patient's bed and the stretcher
   c. Identify the patient
   d. Let the surgeon know that the patient is about to be transferred

7. _____ people should be present during the transfer of a mobile and alert patient.
   a. Two or three
   b. Three or four
   c. Four or five
   d. Five or six

8. The transfer of a conscious patient from a stretcher to an operating table starts with aligning the head of the stretcher with the head of the operating table and then:
   a. Opening up the back of the patient's gown
   b. Identifying the patient
   c. Freeing up the IV tubing
   d. Locking the wheels of the stretcher and the operating room table

9. During the transfer of a conscious patient to the operating room table, the duties of the STSR include:
   a. Protecting the patient's neck and airway
   b. Holding the IV tubing
   c. Controlling the slide board
   d. Nothing, the STSR is preparing the sterile field for surgery and is not needed for assistance during the transfer of a conscious patient to the OR table

10. Position a morbidly obese patient on a _____ surgical table.
   a. Standard
   b. Double
   c. Jackson frame
   d. Bariatric

11. When a patient is placed in the supine position, where is the safety strap placed?
   a. 2 inches below the knees
   b. On the lower abdomen
   c. 2 inches above the knees
   d. On the knees

12. When the patient is positioned in the prone position, the arms should be extended no greater than:
   a. 30 degrees
   b. 60 degrees
   c. 90 degrees
   d. 120 degrees

13. These are used on the patient during surgery to prevent blood pooling and embolism (clot formation):
   a. Bear hugger
   b. Sequential compression device
   c. Hypothermia blanket
   d. Warming blanket

14. The minimum number of people required to perform a lateral transfer of a patient from the stretcher to the operating room table is:
   a. 4
   b. 2
   c. 3
   d. 6

15. Movement of an extremity toward the body is called:
   a. Abduction
   b. Adduction
   c. Circumflexion
   d. Rotation

16. When positioning a pregnant patient, a wedge pad should be placed under the _____ flank to prevent uterine compression on the vena cava, which can cause hypotension and compromise fetal circulation.
   a. Upper thoracic
   b. Left upper thoracic
   c. Right flank
   d. Left buttock

CASE STUDIES

1. *Read the following case study and answer the questions based on your knowledge of patient positioning and use of the operating room table.*

   You have been asked to set up the operating room for a procedure. Today your surgeon will perform a right nephrectomy in operating room 2. The surgeon has told the team that he will be making a flank incision.

   a. In what position will the patient be placed?

b. What position will the patient be in for administration of the general anesthetic?

c. What positioning devices will be needed for this patient?

2. *Read the following case study and answer the questions based on your knowledge of the pregnant patient.*

You are called in for an emergency appendectomy. You are told upon arrival that your patient is pregnant.

a. What position will the patient be placed in?

b. What position devices should you have available?

c. What additional positioning device should be available for positioning your pregnant patient for her appendectomy and why?

17 # Surgical Skin Preparation and Draping

Student's Name _____

KEY TERMS

Write the definition for each term.

1. Antiseptic: _____

2. Debridement: _____

3. Fenestrated drape: _____

4. Impervious: _____

5. Incise drape: _____

6. Residual activity: _____

7. Retention catheter: _____

8. Single-stage prep: _____

9. Solution: _____

10. Squaring the incision: _____

11. Straight catheter: _____

12. Two-stage prep: _____

LABELING

In the drawings below, use a colored pen or pencil to indicate the prep for the procedure listed.

1. Anterior head and neck

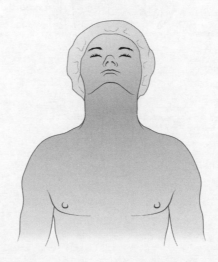

2. Shoulder

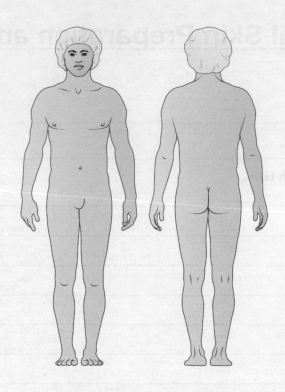

3. Abdomen

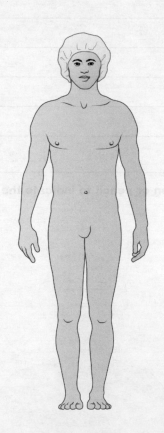

SHORT ANSWERS

Provide a short answer for each question or statement.

1. List the supplies needed for urinary catheterization.

   _____

   _____

2. List the steps of urinary catheterization.

   _____

   _____

3. List the two types of catheterizations and define. List the types of catheters necessary to perform these types of catheterizations.

   _____

   _____

4. What are the CDC guidelines for indications in the operating room for the use of indwelling urethral catheters?

   _____

   _____

5. Antiseptics used for surgical skin prep are mainly evaluated according to what primary criterias?

   _____

   _____

6. Why is iodine a risk of thermal burn when it is heated (warmed)?

   _____

   _____

7. Hair removal requires a verbal or written order by the surgeon. What guidelines should be followed for hair removal?

   _____

   _____

8. The flank and back areas are prepped in the same manner as the abdomen; describe the technique.

   _____

   _____

9. What are the principles of surgical draping?

   _____

   _____

10. List the technique on how to drape equipment such as the operating room microscope.

_____

_____

11. List the sequencing and order of the layers of draping materials used during draping the patient for an abdominal procedure.

_____

_____

12. List the technique in removing drapes.

_____

_____

MATCHING

Match each term with the correct definition. Some terms may be used more than once.

1. _____ destroys microorganisms by *desiccation* (drying) of the cell proteins.

2. _____ has not been approved as a first-choice skin prep by The Joint Commission or CDC.

3. _____ Although it normally is nonirritating to tissue, first-degree and second-degree chemical burns can result from improper prep technique or if the patient is sensitive to iodine.

4. _____ A solution that was removed as a safe skin prep agent. This agent was found to be absorbed through damaged skin of all ages, it was also found to cause damage to the central nervous system in infants.

5. _____ is extremely flammable and volatile.

6. _____ has been linked to hearing loss when accidently introduced in the inner ear.

7. _____ should never be used on mucous membranes or the eyes or in any open wound.

8. _____ should never be used during prep of the eye, ear, or face. Not recommended for use on large open wounds, burns, or infants younger than 2 months of age.

a. Hexachlorophene

b. Iodophors

c. Alcohol 70%

d. Chlorhexidine gluconate (CHG)

MULTIPLE CHOICE

Choose the most correct answer to complete the question or statement.

1. Prewarming a prep solution in a microwave or uncontrolled or unmonitored systems create a risk of:
   a. Allergies
   b. Chemical burn
   c. Fire
   d. Thermal burn

2. Surgical prep agents can cause skin irritation, rash, or other conditions except:
   a. Sterilization of the skin
   b. Chemical and thermal burns
   c. Fire
   d. Allergy

3. Alcohol and alcohol-based prep solutions are volatile and flammable. When alcohol solution or volatile fumes come in contact with heat sources, they can easily cause:
   a. Allergies
   b. Chemical burn
   c. Fire
   d. Thermal burn

4. Serious _____ can occur when prep solutions are allowed to pool under the patient during surgery.
   a. Allergies
   b. Chemical burns
   c. Fires
   d. Thermal burns

5. During the cleansing process, the surgeon removes all foreign material and trims away devitalized tissue called:
   a. Trauma
   b. Cardiac/vascular
   c. Autograft
   d. Debridement

6. _____ is a type of tissue that is removed from one site on the patient and grafted to another site.
   a. Trauma
   b. Cardiac/vascular
   c. Autograft
   d. Debridement

7. _____ wounds are almost always contaminated because they are caused by external forces and often occur in environments that are mildly or grossly contaminated.
   a. Trauma
   b. Cardiac/vascular
   c. Autograft
   d. Debridement

8. _____ require(s) a large area of exposure.
   a. Trauma wounds
   b. Cardiac/vascular inscisions
   c. Autografts
   d. Debridement

9. _____ are folded in a specific way before sterilization so that they can be positioned over the operative site and unfolded in a way that prevents contamination.
   a. Towels
   b. Gowns
   c. Drapes
   d. All the above

10. A retention catheter with a small, inflatable balloon at the tip is called a _____ catheter.
    a. Robinson
    b. Malecot
    c. Fogarty
    d. Foley

11. Catheterization of a female surgical patient requires the _____ position.
    a. Supine
    b. Prone
    c. Lithotomy
    d. Knees slightly flexed

12. Which of the following statements is true regarding the technique for placing a Foley catheter?
    a. The assisting hand does not contact sterile supplies, including the catheter itself.
    b. Both hands must remain sterile for the procedure.
    c. If the catheter is placed before the prep has been done, it is not done using aseptic technique.
    d. The insertion hand does not contact sterile supplies.

13. Healthy skin contains colonies of:
    a. Infection
    b. Bacteria
    c. Grease
    d. Water

14. When is hair removed from the surgical site?
    a. Always
    b. When it will interfere with the procedure, and when the surgeon orders it
    c. When the patient has excess hair
    d. When the patient is a high risk for surgical site infection

15. Which of the following is not true related to performing the surgical prep?
    a. Antiseptic soap solution may be used, followed by a coating of antiseptic solution
    b. Antiseptic solution may be used alone
    c. The prepping agent is selected by the surgeon based on the area to be prepped and any sensitivities the patient may have to prep solutions
    d. The prep used is based on the preferences of the hospital infection control nurse

16. The basic principles of the skin prep:
    a. Is a method to prevent surgical site infection
    b. Is performed prior to draping
    c. Is a method to reduce the number of transient and normal microorganisms to an absolute minimum
    d. All of the above

17. Surgeons apply the surgical drapes in a prescribed order based on:
    a. Aseptic technique
    b. Surgical practice
    c. The patient's risk of infection
    d. Hospital policy

18. To ensure a moisture barrier between the patient and the sterile field, surgical drapes are made of woven and _____ materials.
    a. Polypropylene
    b. Linen
    c. Synthetic
    d. Polyester

19. A draping routine usually begins with:
    a. A plain sheet
    b. A stockinette
    c. A fenestrated drape
    d. A towel or sticky drape

20. The sterile drape that is coated with adhesive on one side and may be impregnated with antiseptic is called a(n):
    a. Three-quarter drape
    b. Fenestrated drape
    c. Half-sheet
    d. Incise drape

21. The procedure drape, or specialty drape, is placed on the patient:
    a. Before the half-sheet
    b. Before the incise drape
    c. First
    d. Last

22. Which of the following rules of asepsis apply to placement of the surgical drapes?
    a. Handle drapes with as much movement as you need to ensure proper placement.
    b. When placing a drape, do not touch the patient's body.
    c. After a drape has been placed, shift or move the drape to make a good fit for the patient and the procedure.
    d. Use perforating towel clips to secure drapes

23. The sterile technique required for catheterization entails application of sterile gloves using open gloving technique and keeping:
    a. Both hands and arms sterile
    b. Both hands unsterile, because this is not a sterile procedure
    c. One hand sterile for insertion of the catheter and using the other gloved hand for exposure of the meatus
    d. Both hands sterile

24. _____ is the most common hospital acquired infection.
    a. Surgical site
    b. Urinary catheterization
    c. Improper prep
    d. All the above

25. Which of the following is recommended to mark the surgical site?
    a. Sharpie
    b. Pen with a ball point
    c. Gentian violet
    d. All of the above

26. Which of the following drapes has a fenestration?
    a. U-drape
    b. Perineal
    c. Utility
    d. Laparotomy

27. How many milliliters of sterile water are required to inflate the 5cc balloon on a Foley catheter?
    a. 5
    b. 10
    c. 7
    d. 6

1. *Read the following case study and answer the questions based on your knowledge of surgical drapes.*

    You are about to scrub for a knee arthroscopy. Your patient is asleep under general anesthesia. He has been prepped, and you are about to drape him. What will you need to have ready for the surgeon so that you can drape the patient? List your supplies in the order you will use them.

18 Surgical Skills I: Planning a Case, Opening, and Start of Surgery

Student's Name _____

KEY TERMS

Write the definition for each term.

1. Blunt dissection: _____

2. Case planning: _____

3. Count: _____

4. Dissecting sponge: _____

5. Event related: _____

6. Graft: _____

7. Implant: _____

8. Radiopaque: _____

9. Raytec: _____

10. Sterile setup: _____

11. Surgeon's preference card: _____

12. TIMEOUT: _____

13. Universal Protocol: _____

SHORT ANSWERS

Provide a short answer for each question or statement.

1. What are the four categories of surgery by objectives?

   a. _____

   b. _____

   c. _____

   d. _____

2. What items are typically found on the surgeon's preference card?

_____

_____

3. What items are included in a surgical count?

_____

_____

4. Who is responsible for ensuring that no item is left in a patient?

_____

_____

5. When are surgical counts performed?

_____

_____

6. Items are usually counted in a specific order; what is that order?

_____

_____

7. Why is a TIMEOUT performed?

_____

_____

8. List synthetic implant materials.

_____

_____

MATCHING

Match each term with the correct description.

1. _____ Means to remove a large portion but not all of a tumor.

2. _____ Separation of one tissue plane from another with use of scissors to increase the space between the layers.

3. _____ Separation of tissue without using sharp instruments.

4. _____ This term means to carefully separate anatomical structures by cutting with instruments, small firm sponges, or the fingers.

5. _____ Enable precise reviewing of an anatomical area.

6. _____ This term usually refers to the removal of a limb or digit.

7. _____ To constrict a vessel or duct using a suture tie.

8. _____ This refers to the joining of two hollow anatomical structures (vessels, ducts, tubes, or hollow organs) using sutures or surgical staples.

9. _____ The use of sharp surgical instruments such as a scalpel and scissors to cut away dead tissue.

10. _____ The spaces and tissues that are accessed through the surgical incision.

11. _____ To bring a tissue structure partially outside the body.

12. _____ To raise or lift an anatomical structure, sometimes without removing it.

13. _____ A large portion or segment of tissue is removed.

14. _____ The removal of tissue, usually a mole or small lesion using cutting instruments or electrosurgery.

15. _____ The sterile area immediately around or in the surgical incision.

16. _____ This refers to an undesirable pucker in skin as a result of poor suture placement.

17. _____ In surgical terms, this means to "bring together" tissues by suturing or other means.

a. Amputate

b. Anastomose

c. Approximate

d. Blunt dissection

e. Debridement

f. Dog ear

g. Debulk

h. Dissect

i. Elevate

j. Excise

k. Exposure

l. Exteriorize

m. Ligate

n. Resection

o. Surgical field

p. Surgical wound

q. Undermine

MATCHING

Match each term with the correct definition as it applies to implants and grafts.

1. _____ Tissue used to cover large defects in the skin.

2. _____ Graft made from nonliving cadaver bone.

3. _____ Grafts made from a combination of cadaver bone, morcellated allograft bone and marrow.

4. _____ Used as a biological dressing for burns, skin ulcers, and infected wounds.

5. _____ Any type of tissue replacement or device placed in the body.

6. _____ Tissue graft derived from human tissue.

7. _____ Graft taken from pig tissue.

8. _____ Tissue obtained from the patient's body and implanted in another site.

9. _____ Graft taken from a species different from that of the patient.

10. _____ Migration of epithelial cells into the wound during healing.

11. _____ Graft taken from beef origin.

a. Allogeneic graft

b. Allograft

c. Amniotic membrane and unbilical cord

d. Autograft

e. Bovine graft

f. Composite graft

g. Epithelialization

h. Implant

i. Porcine graft

j. Xenograft

k. Wound cover

MULTIPLE CHOICE

Choose the most correct answer to complete the question or statement.

1. Case planning combines knowledge of:
   a. Surgical procedure and surgical techniques
   b. Anatomy and pathology
   c. The patient's diagnosis
   d. The patient's prognosis

2. When opening packages sealed with tape, why should you break the tape rather than peel the tape off?
   a. To prevent the outer wrapper from ripping, causing contamination
   b. So that you have to look at the tape to see whether it is sterile
   c. To prevent strike-through
   d. To prevent the inner wrapper from ripping

3. Which of the following is *not* a recommendation for opening a case?
   a. Open the scrubbed surgical technologist's gown and gloves on a small table or Mayo stand.
   b. Never unwrap a heavy item by holding it in midair.
   c. Do not open small sterile items into the genesis instrument tray.
   d. Open extra sutures, special equipment, and implants so that the surgeon does not have to wait for them during the procedure.

4. After the case has been opened, the surgical technologist's next immediate task is to:
   a. Load the knife blade
   b. Dress the Mayo stand
   c. Perform a surgical hand scrub
   d. Organize the instruments

5. Using a methodical method for all sterile set-ups in the learning stages:
   a. Makes the instruments easy for the surgeon to reach
   b. Contaminates the back table
   c. Improves efficiency and decreases great stress and errors
   d. Is against the Association of Perioperative Registered Nurses (AORN) standards

6. After finishing the surgical scrub, which task is done next?
   a. Arrange towels, gowns, and gloves in order of use
   b. Gown and glove self
   c. Organize the knife and the instruments
   d. Put all sponges in one location so you are ready to count

7. The selection of suture material is almost always prescriptive, or:
   a. Written on the surgeon's case plan ahead of time
   b. Delayed until the surgeon can prescribe the type she wants
   c. Determined only after the surgeon has taken a look at the surgical wound
   d. Delayed until the surgeon has discussed surgical wound closure with the patient.

8. If the count is incorrect:
   a. A radiograph should be taken immediately.
   b. The surgeon should not be bothered.
   c. The surgeon is notified and the count repeated.
   d. The circulator should call the house supervisor for an incident report.

9. A retained item can cause patient injury from all of the following, *except*:
   a. X-ray exposure sickness
   b. Infection
   c. Organ perforation
   d. Obstruction

10. Immediately after gowning and gloving, the technologist must complete:
    a. Scattering the case
    b. The sterile setup or setting up a case
    c. Preparation of the operating room
    d. The surgical count

11. After you scrub and as you first approach the pile of sterile equipment, do not move anything until:
    a. You have a plan
    b. You count the instruments
    c. You load the blade on the knife handle
    d. You move the drapes and put them in order

12. Tissue derived from human tissue acquired from a tissue bank is called:
    a. Allograft
    b. Synthetic implant
    c. Autologous autograft
    d. Silicone

13. Tissue obtained from the patient's own body, implanted into another site, is called:
    a. Allograft
    b. Silicone
    c. Synthetic implant
    d. Autologous autograft

CASE STUDIES

1. *Read the following case study and answer the questions based on your knowledge of case preparation.*

   It is 6:30 AM, and you are assigned to operating room 6 with your preceptor, who has called and said that she will be late because she has a flat tire. She has asked that you go ahead and get the room ready for the day, "pick the case," and then place the sterile unopened packs onto the furniture where they will be opened soon. She does not want you to "open the case" until she gets there to assist you. How should you proceed?

Surgical Skills II: Intraoperative and Immediate Postoperative Period

Student's Name _____

KEY TERMS _____

Write the definition for each term.

1. Absorbable suture: _____

2. Adhesion: _____

3. Anastomosis: _____

4. Approximate: _____

5. Biopsy: _____

6. Capillary action: _____

7. Dehiscence: _____

8. Detachable suture: _____

9. Evisceration: _____

10. Frozen section: _____

11. Hematoma: _____

12. Hemostasis: _____

13. Inert: _____

14. Interrupted sutures: _____

15. Nonabsorbable suture: _____

16. Primary intention: _____

17. Reverse cutting needle: _____

18. Swage: _____

19. Tensile strength: _____

20. Tie on a passer: _____

SHORT ANSWERS

Provide a short answer for each question or statement.

1. List types of surgical sponges and their uses that are commonly used in the operating room.

   _____

   _____

   _____

   _____

   _____

   _____

2. List Halstead's principles of surgery and define.

   1. _____

   2. _____

   3. _____

   4. _____

   5. _____

   6. _____

   7. _____

3. What are the primary techniques of hemostasis used in surgery?

   a. _____

   b. _____

   c. _____

   d. _____

4. What are the three categories of physical structures of sutures?

   1. _____

   2. _____

   2a. _____

   2b. _____

   3. _____

Chapter **19** **Surgical Skills II: Intraoperative and Immediate Postoperative Period**

5. List classifications of wounds and provice characteristics and examples of each.

1. _____

2. _____

3. _____

4. _____

6. All substances, including suture products, that bear the USP label must meet minimum standards. What are the standards for sutures?

_____

_____

7. List the physical characteristics of sutures that influence a surgeon's decision in choosing a suture.

1. _____

2. _____

3. _____

4. _____

5. _____

6. _____

7. _____

8. _____

9. _____

10. _____

8. List materials that are the most inert in tissue.

_____

_____

9. Describe the types of suture needles.

_____

_____

10. List important considerations that may determine which type of suture is selected to be used in particular tissues.

_____

_____

_____

_____

_____

_____

11. What are the purposes of wound dressings?

_____

_____

LABELING

Label the following pictures with the type of suture technique shown.

1. _____

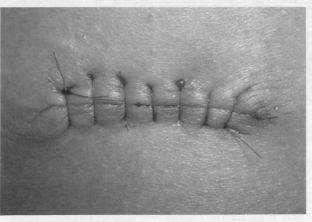

2. _____

Chapter **19** Surgical Skills II: Intraoperative and Immediate Postoperative Period

3. _____

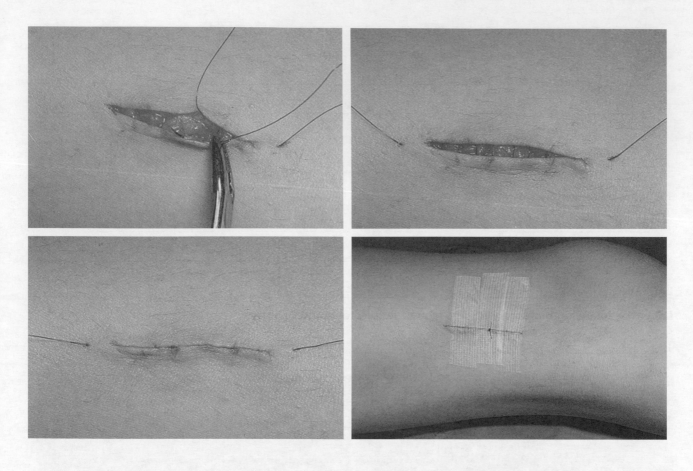

4. _____

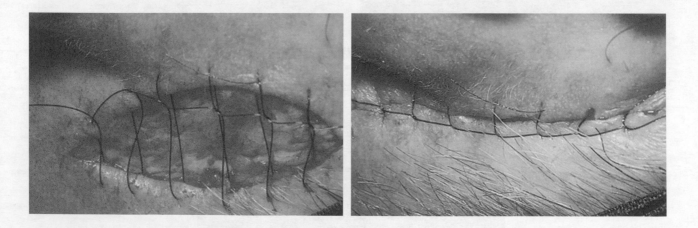

5. _____

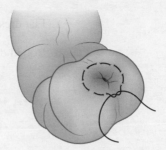

6. _____

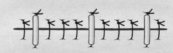

MATCHING I

Match the wound drains to the category of wound drainage system

1. _____ Jackson Pratt   a. Passive drain

2. _____ Malecot   b. Suction drain

3. _____ Penrose   c. Water-sealed drainage system

4. _____ Stoma pouch   d. Collection of body fluids from an artificial orifice

5. _____ Pezzar

6. _____ Chest drainage tubes

7. _____ Hemovac

MATCHING II

Match the following dressings

1. _____ ABD pad

2. _____ Tube stockinet

3. _____ Telfa

4. _____ Coban

5. _____ Adaptic - petroleum based agent

6. _____ Elastoplast

7. _____ 4 x 4 gauze sponges

8. _____ Kling gauze

a. Flat dressing

b. Rolled dressing

MATCHING III

Match the following wound complications

1. _____ Tissue breakdown at the edges of the wound causing the wound edges to open up

2. _____ Bands of scar tissue in the abdominal area, pelvic organs, and peritoneum

3. _____ Usually occurs during the first week post op beginning with an excess of inflammation and serious discharge from the wound

4. _____ collection of blood that forms in a wound due to incomplete hemostasis or capillary bleeding

5. _____ tissue breakdown of the wound with protrusion of the abdominal contents outside of the wound, can involve the omentum and or bowel

6. _____ Collection of fluid that develops in the wound during healing caused by tissue trauma incurred during the procedure, acting as a physical barrier between the wound edges preventing healing

a. Surgical site infection

b. Seroma

c. Hematoma

d. Dehiscence

e. Evisceration

f. Adhesions

MULTIPLE CHOICE

Choose the most correct answer to complete the question or statement.

1. Which of the following specimens might be sent to the pathologist on a Telfa sponge?
   a. Adenoid tissue
   b. Prostate from a transurethral resection of the prostate (TURP)
   c. Uterus and fallopian tubes
   d. Breast tissue for frozen section

2. Which of the following specimens must be sent to the pathologist dry?
   a. Colon polyps
   b. Bronchial washings
   c. Kidney stones
   d. Tonsils

3. Which sponge is used to make a sponge stick?
   a. Laparotomy
   b. Raytec
   c. Kittner
   d. Tonsil

4. Which type of sponge is packaged in groups of 10?
   a. Kittner
   b. Cherry
   c. Raytec
   d. Laparotomy

5. Which type of sponge would be appropriate for "packing" the abdominal cavity?
   a. Kittner
   b. Raytec
   c. Laparotomy
   d. Neuro patties

6. Uncontrolled oozing or insecure hemostasis can lead to a:
   a. Hematoma
   b. Contusion
   c. Seroma
   d. Compartment syndrome

7. Tissue breakdown at the wound margins which causes the wound to open up is called:
   a. Evisceration
   b. Adhesions
   c. Dehiscence
   d. Hematoma

8. Suture materials are used for all of the following, *except:*
   a. Approximation
   b. Ligation of tubular structures
   c. Hemostasis
   d. Coagulation

9. Which of the following is the *largest* suture?
   a. # 1 Ethibond
   b. # 0 silk
   c. 3-0 Vicryl
   d. 11-0 chromic

10. The physical characteristics of a suture include which of the following?
    a. Size
    b. Elasticity
    c. Memory
    d. Effect of the suture on the tissue

11. A bridal suture used in ophthalmic surgery is also called a(an):
    a. Retention suture
    b. Subcutaneous suture
    c. Traction suture
    d. Vertical mattress suture

12. The _____ of suture refers to the amount of force needed to break the suture.
    a. Knot strength
    b. Tensile strength
    c. Tissue drag
    d. Biological environment

13. Sutures made of multifilament strands can hold body fluids which can retain and carry infections by the sutures by:
    a. Osmosis
    b. Wicking or capillary action
    c. Monofilament
    d. Inert

14. A wound that is not sutured and must heal from the base is healing by: _____
    a. Delayed union
    b. First intention
    c. Secondary intention
    d. Third intention

15. Which of the following is the first phase of wound healing?
    a. Healing phase
    b. Remodeling phase
    c. Proliferative phase
    d. Inflammatory phase

16. Which of the following is *not* considered a risk factor in wound healing?
    a. Nutritional status
    b. Chronic disease
    c. Obesity
    d. Healthy 20-year-old athlete

17. Which type of sponge is used in neurosurgical procedures?
    a. Pusher
    b. Kitner
    c. Laparotomy
    d. Cottonoid

18. Which type of sponge is used for blunt dissection?
    a. Cottonoid
    b. Peanut
    c. Tonsil
    d. Patty

19. Removal of an entire mass of suspicious area of tissue:
    a. Core needle biopsy
    b. Fine needle aspiration
    c. Excisional biopsy
    d. Incisional biopsy

20. Tissue biopsy with use of a long fine needle to aspirate small pieces of tissue:
    a. Core needle biopsy
    b. Fine needle aspiration
    c. Excisional biopsy
    d. Incisional biopsy

21. Tissue biopsy with use of a large bore hollow trocar or needle:
   a. Core needle biopsy
   b. Fine needle aspiration
   c. Excisional biopsy
   d. Incisional biopsy

22. Partial removal of a tissue mass:
   a. Core needle biopsy
   b. Fine needle aspiration
   c. Excisional biopsy
   d. Incisional biopsy

23. Immediate analysis of tissue for malignancy is called a frozen section, the tissue is sent to the pathology department:
   a. In Normal Saline solution
   b. Fresh with no fixative
   c. In Formalin
   d. In sterile water

24. When handling forensic evidence such as bullets how should you handle the item?
   a. Handle item with hemostatic forceps
   b. Handle item with tooth forceps
   c. Handle item carefully to avoid scratching or distorting
   d. Send the item to pathology

25. Which type of needle is used on the liver?
   a. Cutting
   b. Blunt
   c. Taper
   d. Taper cut

26. Which type of needle would be used on soft tissues such as the gastrointestinal tissue?
   a. Cutting
   b. Blunt
   c. Taper
   d. Reverse cutting

27. Which type of needle would be used on tendons or skin?
   a. Cutting
   b. Blunt
   c. Taper
   d. Spatula

28. Which type of suture is used to provide additional support to wound edges?
   a. Retention
   b. Vertical mattress
   c. Horizontal mattress
   d. Purse-string

29. Commonly called a stick tie:
   a. Tie on a passer
   b. Free tie
   c. Suture ligature
   d. Reel

CASE STUDIES

1. *You have been precepting new students in the operating room and know how challenging it is to learn sutures. You want to create something to simplify the process of learning sutures. You decide you are going to make a suture square:*

   Using the squares below, categorize the sutures from the text. After you have finished that, use a colored pencil to make the suture name in the same color as the suture package.

	Synthetic Sutures	Natural Sutures
Absorbable sutures		
Nonabsorbable sutures		

20 Minimally Invasive Surgery

Student's Name _____

KEY TERMS

Write the definition for each term.

1. Active electrode monitoring (AEM): _____

2. Arthroscopy: _____

3. Auxiliary water channel: _____

4. Biopsy channel: _____

5. Camera control unit (CCU): _____

6. Cannula: _____

7. Capacitative coupling: _____

8. Control head: _____

9. Direct coupling: _____

10. Elevator channel: _____

11. Endocoupler: _____

12. Gain: _____

13. High definition (HD): _____

14. Imaging system: _____

15. Insertion tube: _____

16. Instrument channel: _____

17. Insufflation: _____

18. Intravasation: _____

19. Light cable: _____

20. Light source: _____

21. Optical angle: _____

22. Pixel: _____

23. Pneumoperitoneum: _____

24. Port: _____

25. Resectoscope: _____

26. Standard definition (SD): _____

27. White balance: _____

SHORT ANSWER

Provide a short answer for each question or statement.

1. Describe the difference between rigid endoscopy and flexible endoscopy.

   _____

   _____

2. What are the special considerations when prepping and draping for MIS procedures?

   _____

   _____

3. What are the components of the surgical imaging system?

   _____

   _____

4. The guidelines for taking care of the fiberoptic cables include:

   a. _____

   b. _____

   c. _____

   d. _____

   e. _____

   f. _____

   g. _____

5. What is the procedure for white balancing?

   _____

   _____

6. Describe the process of insufflation.

   _____

   _____

7. What is the procedure for insertion of a Veress needle?

_____

_____

8. What is the purpose of continuous irrigation and fluid distension? Which types of procedures is it commonly used during?

_____

_____

MATCHING

Match each term with the correct definition. You may use the same answer more than once.

1. _____ In minimally invasive surgery, the inflation of the abdominal or thoracic cavity with carbon dioxide gas.

2. _____ Refers to the abdomen when it is distended with carbon dioxide gas.

3. _____ A trocar that is rounded at the tip.

4. _____ In MIS suturing and knot tying, technique performed "inside the body."

5. _____ A device that controls and emits light for delivery in endoscopic procedures.

6. _____ A sharp, rod-shaped instrument used to puncture the body wall.

7. _____ Connects the camera to the telescope.

8. _____ Long, narrow instruments with an optical lens used during endoscopic surgery.

9. _____ A hollow tube that holds the trocar.

10. _____ A spring-loaded needle used to deliver carbon dioxide gas during insufflation.

11. _____ The suture or pre-tied loop used when a tissue structure requires ligation rather than suturing.

12. _____ The fiberoptic light cable that transmits light from the source to the endoscopic instrument.

13. _____ Refers to the rigid lensed instrument used in minimally invasive surgery.

14. _____ Instrument passed through a natural orifice for assessment or surgery of a hollow organ, duct, or vessel performed with a flexible, semi-rigid or rigid endoscope.

a. Light source

b. Light cable

c. Endoscope

d. Cannula

e. Blunt trocar

f. Telescopic instruments

g. Intracorporeal

h. Veress needle

i. Insufflation

j. Pneumoperitoneum

k. Trocar

l. Ligation loop

m. Endocoupler

Title Match the parts of a flexible endoscope

_____1. Receives the biopsy forceps, brushes, and other instruments used to obtain specimens

_____2. Connects with the digital camera, optical system control handles, suction and irrigation

_____3. Used to insufflate the lumen of the gastrointestinal tract to create space in the same way as a pneumoperitoneum

_____4. Port located near the junction of the control head and insertion tube

_____5. Channel used to clear blood and tissue debris from the lens

_____6. Component of the endoscope that enters the patient's body

a. Air channel

b. Auxillary water channel

c. Biopsy channel

d. Instrument channel

e. Insertion tube

f. Control head

MULTIPLE CHOICE

1. Patient position for laparoscopic procedures of the upper abdomen and lower esophagus is:
   a. Reverse Trendelenburg
   b. Beach chair
   c. Semi fowlers
   d. Trendelenburg

2. Patient position for laparoscopic procedures of the lower abdomen and pelvis is:
   a. Jack knife
   b. Trendelenburg
   c. Reverse Trendelenburg
   d. Kraske

3. Patient position for laparoscopic procedures of the shoulder is:
   a. Trendelenburg
   b. Beach chair
   c. Decubitis
   d. Lateral decubitis

4. Patient position for video-assisted thorascopic procedures is:
   a. Supine
   b. Prone
   c. Beach chair
   d. Lateral decubitis

CASE STUDIES

1. _You are scrubbed in on a laparoscopic procedure that is about to finish. Your responsibility as a surgical technologist is to properly handle and care for the laparoscope in a manner that prevents damage. What does that include?_

   a. _____

   b. _____

c. _____

d. _____

e. _____

2. *During a laparoscopic procedure an emergency situation occurs, and the surgeon needs to convert to an open procedure. What will the process be while you are converting to an open case?*

a. _____

b. _____

c. _____

d. _____

e. _____

f. _____

21 Robotic-Assisted Surgery

Student's Name _____

KEY TERMS

Write the definition for each term.

1. Bedside unit: _____

_____

2. Docking: _____

_____

3. Hand controllers: _____

_____

4. Haptic feedback (force pressure): _____

_____

5. Modular robotic system: _____

_____

6. Near-infrared imaging: _____

_____

7. Port: _____

_____

8. Registration (of a digital image): _____

_____

9. Remote data display: _____

_____

10. Reposable: _____

_____

11. Robotic-assisted surgical system (RAS): _____

_____

12. Scaled movement: _____

_____

13. Surgeon console: _____

_____

14. Surgical access: _____

15. Wristed instruments: _____

_____

SHORT ANSWER

Provide a short answer for each question or statement.

1. Robotic-assisted surgery evolved from the technology of minimally invasive surgery. Describe the similarities.

_____

_____

_____

_____

_____

_____

2. What does the U.S Food and Drug Administration define robotic-assisted surgical device as a subtype of?

_____

_____

3. Differentiate between the Veress needle technique and Hasson techniques for creation of pneumoperitoneum.

_____

_____

_____

_____

_____

MATCHING I

Match each term with the correct definition.

1. _____ Accessory equipment tower in which equipment such as energy modalities, system electronics, video controller, and touch screen are placed where signals relayed by fiber optic cables to the surgeon console can be controlled.

2. _____ Refers to providing sense of touch.

3. _____ Freely moveable unit system that features a single instrument and its arm that is attached to a dedicated base.

4. _____ Nonsterile control station where the surgeon sits or stands while operating.

5. _____ CT or MRI scans can be displayed on the screen monitor at any time.

6. _____ Describes instruments that feature a long shaft, working tip, and head that attaches to the robotic arm.

7. _____ Used to move the surgical instruments during the procedure.

8. _____ Provides three-dimensional images, as well as an endoscopic field of vision that can be panned or out without loss of image, quality, or light.

9. _____ Refers to the tips of the robotic instruments in a nose-up and nose-down position.

10. _____ Surgeon console system referred to as immersive featuring a cockpit-style viewer.

11. _____ Used on some systems to activate the energy instruments.

12. _____ Surgeon console system that has no cockpit or hood.

13. _____ Refers to the tips of the robotic instruments making right and left turns in a space.

14. _____ Receptacle for the surgical instruments and endoscope that are inserted into designated arms.

a. Surgeon console

b. Open console design

c. Closed console design

d. Remote data display

e. Hand controllers

f. Foot controls

g. Bedside unit

h. Modular robotic system

i. Optics

j. Vision tower

k. Wristed

l. *Pitch*

m. *Yaw*

n. Haptic

Match each type or robotic system with the correct definition.

_____ 1. Robotically controlled bronchoscope with a high degree of flexibility and high-definition 3-D vision used during bronchoscopy for taking biopsies and some therapeutic procedures.

_____ 2. A modular system with freely moveable bedside carts for each instrument and the endoscope. It is a robotic-assisted digital system featuring an open surgeon console and uses standard, reusable, minimally invasive instruments and trocar-cannula systems.

_____ 3. System features modular, freely moveable bedside carts for wristed instruments and the robotic endoscope providing 3-D viewing and motionless endoscopic field of vision. The surgical non-haptic instruments are reposable, and the system uses compatible energy devices.

_____ 4. Semi-robotic platform that features a flexible endoscope and robotically controlled instruments commonly used in transoral and transanal surgical procedures.

_____ 5. System has a closed surgeon console, single bedside cart with multiple instrument arms mounted on a central column, robotic endoscope, and 3-D viewing. Instrumentation is reposable, the system does not have haptic feedback.

_____ 6. Orthopedic robotic-assistive system used to enable accurate bone preparation and tissue balancing for total or partial joint replacement.

a. Versius (CMR Surgical)

b. daVinci

c. Senhance

d. Joint arthroplasty system

e. Flex Robotic (Medrobotics, Inc.)

f. Monarch Platform (Auris Health)

MULTIPLE CHOICE

1. Cause of conversion from a robotic case to an open case is:
   a. Loss of vision
   b. Instrument failure
   c. Hemorrhage
   d. All of the above

2. After placing the Veress needle, why is a small amount of saline lightly injected or dropped into the needle hub?
   a. To create negative pressure
   b. To create pneumoperitoneum
   c. If the saline flows, the Veress needle is in proper placement
   d. If the saline does not flow, it means the Veress needle is in proper placement

3. Robotic team member responsible for direct patient care, protecting the sterile field, assisting the anesthesia provider, and assisting in setting up the robotic equipment and driving the base unit or patient cart into place:
   a. Assistant surgeon
   b. Circulating nurse
   c. Surgical technologist
   d. Robotics coordinator

4. What type of serious complications can pneumoperitoneum cause related to anesthesia during the procedure?
   a. Decreased lung capacity
   b. Increased body temperature
   c. Increased lung capacity
   d. Decreased body temperature

1. *You are assigned to scrub in the robotics room. What are the steps in preoperative preparation as well as the initial setup of the sterile field and start of surgery?*

22 General Surgery

Student's Name _____

KEY TERMS

Write the definition for each term associated with the abdomen.

1. Abdominal peritoneum: _____

2. Adhesions: _____

3. Direct inguinal repair: _____

4. Fistula: _____

5. Hernia: _____

6. Incarcerated hernia: _____

7. Incisional hernia: _____

8. Indirect inguinal hernia: _____

9. Linea alba: _____

10. McBurney incision: _____

11. Resection: _____

12. Ventral hernia: _____

13. Viscera: _____

Write the definition for each term associated with the bowel.

1. Anastomosis: _____

2. Billroth I procedure: _____

3. Billroth II procedure: _____

4. Exploratory laparotomy: _____

5. Gastrostomy: _____

6. Isolation technique: _____

7. Laparotomy: _____

8. Morbid obesity: _____

9. -ostomy: _____

142

10. Stoma: _____

11. Stoma appliance: _____

Write the definition for each term associated with the liver and spleen.

1. Cirrhosis: _____

2. Lobectomy: _____

3. Segmental resection: _____

Write the definition for each term associated with the breast.

1. Body image: _____

2. Needle wire localization: _____

3. Mastectomy: _____

4. Modified radical mastectomy: _____

5. Sentinel lymph node biopsy (SLNB): _____

6. Skin flap: _____

7. Subcutaneous mastectomy: _____

8. Technetium-99: _____

Label the axillary anatomy of the breast.

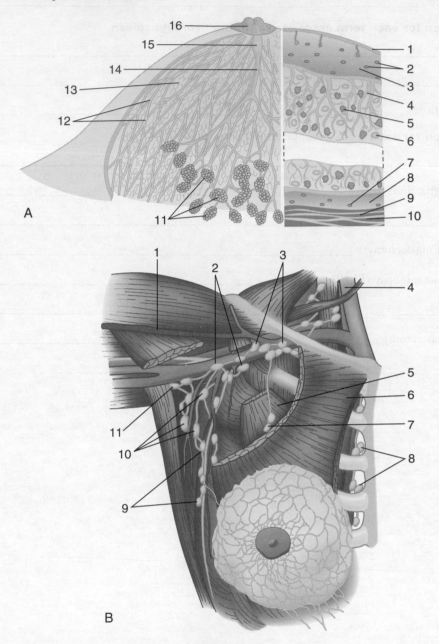

A.

1. _____

2. _____

3. _____

4. _____

5. _____

6. _____

7. _____

8. _____

9. _____

10. _____

11. _____

12. _____

13. _____

14. _____

15. _____

16. _____

B. 1. _____

2. _____

3. _____

4. _____

5. _____

6. _____

7. _____

8. _____

9. _____

10. _____

11. _____

Chapter **22** **General Surgery**

Label the biliary and hepatic anatomy.

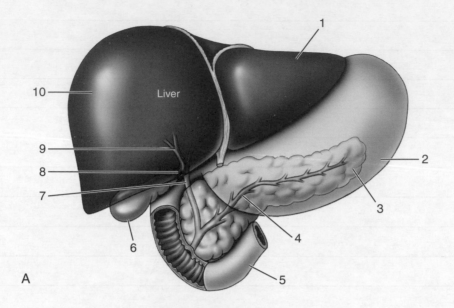

A

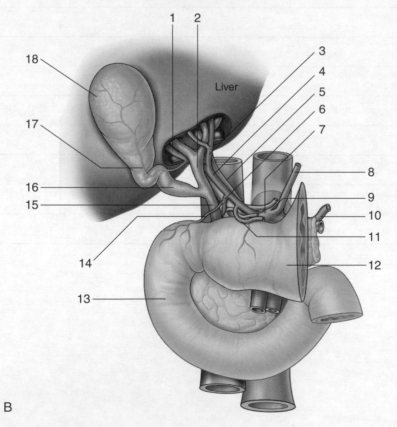

B

A. 1. _____
   2. _____
   3. _____
   4. _____
   5. _____
   6. _____
   7. _____
   8. _____
   9. _____
   10. _____

B. 1. _____
   2. _____
   3. _____
   4. _____
   5. _____
   6. _____
   7. _____
   8. _____
   9. _____
   10. _____
   11. _____
   12. _____
   13. _____
   14. _____
   15. _____
   16. _____
   17. _____
   18. _____

Draw in the following types of abdominal incisions.

1. Subcostal

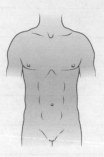

2. Paramedian

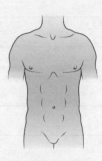

3. McBurney

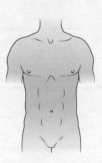

4. Pfannenstiel

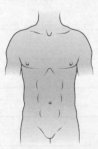

5. Upper midline

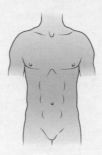

6. Upper abdominal transverse

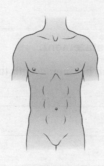

7. Oblique

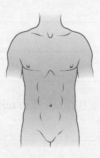

8. Lower midline

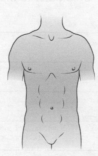

9. Draw the four quadrants of the abdomen and label them.

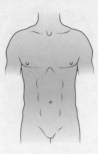

SHORT ANSWER

Provide a short answer for each question or statement.

1. List the three anatomical sections of the stomach beginning with the upper portion.

    a. _____

    b. _____

    c. _____

2. What are the components of the Hesselbach triangle?

    a. _____

    b. _____

    c. _____

3. What is the difference between a Billroth I and a Billroth II in terms of resection and anastomosis?

    _____

    _____

4. What are the tissue layers of the abdominal wall from outer to inner?

    a. _____

    b. _____

    c. _____

    d. _____

    e. _____

5. What are the layers of the intestine from inner to outer?

    a. _____

    b. _____

    c. _____

6. Define the following intestinal conditions.

   a. Volvulus: _____

   b. Intussusception: _____

   c. Paralytic ileus: _____

   d. Peptic ulcer: _____

7. Define the following endoscopic procedures, and what organs are being viewed for diagnosis.

   1. EGD: _____

   2. Colonoscopy: _____

   3. Sigmoidoscopy: _____

   4. ERCP: _____

   5. Choledochoscopy: _____

MATCHING I

Match each term with the correct definition.

1. _____ Hernia that results from a defect in the inguinal floor. The defect is located in the Hesselbach triangle.

2. _____ Herniated tissue that is trapped in an abdominal wall defect causing loss of blood supply.

3. _____ A tract or tunnel through the tissue developing an epithelial lining preventing the wound from healing in an incisional hernia.

4. _____ Abdominal wall defect occurring in the linea alba at the umbilical ring.

5. _____ Postoperative herniation of tissue into the tissue layers of an abdominal incision.

6. _____ Hernia protrusion of the abdominal viscera into the inguinal canal from the deep inguinal ring.

7. _____ Hernia in which abdominal tissue has become trapped or strangulated by surrounding tissue between the layers of an abdominal wall defect.

8. _____ A type of incisional hernia.

9. _____ Rare hernia that occurs between the transverse abdominis and rectus muscles.

a. Ventral hernia

b. Direct inguinal hernia

c. Incisional hernia

d. Incarcerated hernia

e. Umbilical

f. Fistula

g. Indirect inguinal hernia

h. Strangulated hernia

i. Spigelian

MATCHING II

Match each type of breast procedure with the correct definition.

1. _____ Removal of a wire localized tissue mass for pathologic examination.

2. _____ The entire breast is removed and sentinel node biopsy or axillary dissection is performed.

3. _____ Removal of a breast mass ensuring margins are completely free of cancer cells. Axillary node dissection may be performed at the same time.

4. _____ Procedure in which a hook wire device is inserted into a breast mass using guided imagery.

5. _____ Procedure that removes the breast while leaving the skin, nipple, and areola intact.

6. _____ Skin sparing procedure in which one or more lymph nodes are removed to determine whether a tumor has metastasized; nodes are identified by isosulfan blue dye or technetium-99.

7. _____ Procedure that removes breast tissue, including the skin, areola, and nipple. The axillary lymph nodes are not removed.

8. _____ The entire breast, all axillary nodes, and chest wall muscles are removed.

a. Wire localization

b. Excisional biopsy

c. Lumpectomy

d. Radical mastectomy

e. Modified radical mastectomy

f. Sentinel lymph node biopsy

g. Simple mastectomy

h. Subcutaneous mastectomy

MATCHING III

Match the portions of the gastrointestinal tract.

1. _____ 10-inch tubular structure extending from the pharynx to the stomach entering the abdominal cavity at the diaphragm.

2. _____ The first portion of the large intestine.

3. _____ The distal 4 to 5 inches of the intestine.

4. _____ Extends from the distal ileum to the rectum and is divided into five sections.

5. _____ Area where muscular sphincters control the release of feces.

6. _____ Slender worm-shaped tube at the terminal end of the cecum that has no function.

7. _____ The first portion of the small intestine.

8. _____ The second portion of the small intestine.

9. _____ Sphincter that communicates the stomach with the esophagus.

10. _____ Connects to the esophagus containing the fundus, body, and antrum.

11. _____ The area where the rectum terminates.

12. _____ The distal portion of the small intestine connecting to the large intestine.

a. Jejunum

b. Pylorus

c. Rectum

d. Anal canal

e. Esophagus

f. Stomach

g. Cecum

h. Veriform appendix

i. Large intestine

j. Ileum

k. Cardia

l. Anal canal

152

MULTIPLE CHOICE

1. Removal of the entire breast, all axillary nodes, and chest wall muscles is called:
   a. Lumpectomy
   b. Sentinel lymph node biopsy
   c. Modified radical mastectomy
   d. Radical mastectomy

2. Injection of dye or radioactive material to provide visibility of nodes for removal is called:
   a. Lumpectomy
   b. Sentinel lymph node biopsy
   c. Modified radical mastectomy
   d. Radical mastectomy

3. Removal of a breast mass to confirm a diagnosis or to treat malignancy is called:
   a. Radical mastectomy
   b. Modified radical mastectomy
   c. Lumpectomy
   d. Sentinel lymph node biopsy

4. Removal of the entire breast and sentinel node biopsy or performing axillary dissection is called:
   a. Radical mastectomy
   b. Modified radical mastectomy
   c. Lumpectomy
   d. Sentinel lymph node biopsy

5. During a cholecystectomy, what is ligated?
   a. Common bile duct and cystic artery
   b. Common bile duct and cystic duct
   c. Cystic duct and cystic artery
   d. Common bile duct and common bile artery

6. During a cholecystectomy, which is preserved?
   a. Cystic duct
   b. Common bile duct
   c. Cystic artery
   d. Common bile artery

7. Which of the following is the procedure to treat gastroesophageal reflux disease (GERD)?
   a. Lap band gastroplasty
   b. Roux-en-y gastric bypass
   c. Nissen fundoplication
   d. Laparotomy

8. Which of the following procedures is performed to treat cancer of the head of the pancreas?
   a. Billroth I
   b. LeFort I
   c. Billroth II
   d. Whipple

9. Insulin and glucagon are synthesized in the region of the pancreas called:
   a. Islets of Langerhans
   b. Pancreatic duct
   c. Sphincter of Wirsung
   d. Ampulla of Vater

10. Bile enters the duodenum through an opening called:
    a. Islets of Langerhans
    b. Pancreatic duct
    c. Duct of Wirsung
    d. Ampulla of Vater

11. The release of bile and pancreatic enzymes is controlled by a sphincter in the ampulla called the sphincter of:
    a. Wirsung
    b. Odi
    c. Vater
    d. Langerhans

CASE STUDIES

1. *You are scrubbed in on an emergency endoscopic appendectomy. What are the steps (in order) for performing an appendectomy?*

_____

23 Gynecological and Obstetrical Surgery

Student's Name _____

Write the definition for each term associated with gynecology and reproduction.

1. Ablate: _____

2. Adnexa: _____

3. Coitus: _____

4. Colposcopy: _____

5. Cystocele: _____

6. Dermoid cyst: _____

7. Electrolytic fluid: _____

8. Episiotomy: _____

9. Fibroid: _____

10. Hyperplasia: _____

11. Incomplete abortion: _____

12. LEEP: _____

13. Leiomyoma: _____

14. Menarche: _____

15. Menorrhagia: _____

16. Missed abortion: _____

17. Obturator: _____

18. Papanicolaou (Pap) test: _____

19. Parturition: _____

20. Perineum: _____

21. PID: _____

22. Transcervical: _____

Write the definition for each term associated with obstetrics.

23. Amniotic fluid: _____

24. Amniotic membranes: _____

25. Apgar score: _____

26. Birth canal: _____

27. Breech presentation: _____

28. Cerclage: _____

29. Cord prolapse: _____

30. Eclampsia: _____

31. Ectopic pregnancy: _____

32. Epidural: _____

33. Fetal demise: _____

34. Gestational age: _____

35. Incompetent cervix: _____

36. Labor: _____

37. Meconium: _____

38. Normal spontaneous vaginal delivery: _____

39. Nuchal cord: _____

40. Placenta: _____

41. Placental abruption: _____

42. Placenta previa: _____

43. Prenatal: _____

44. Presentation: _____

45. STD: _____

46. Suprapubic pressure: _____

47. Uterus: _____

LABELING

Label the structures of the vulva.

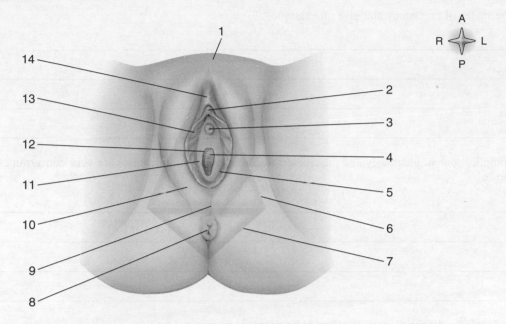

From Thibodeau G, Patton K: *Anatomy and physiology*, ed 6, St Louis, 2007, Mosby.

1. _____
2. _____
3. _____
4. _____
5. _____
6. _____
7. _____
8. _____
9. _____
10. _____
11. _____
12. _____
13. _____
14. _____

Provide a short answer for each question or statement.

1. Explain the stages of pregnancy and give an example.

   _____

   _____

   _____

   _____

2. List the complications of pregnancy and provide details on why the complications are very concerning for the mother and baby.

   _____

   _____

   _____

   _____

3. List the gynecologic diagnostic tests performed on pregnant women.

   _____

   _____

   _____

   _____

4. What is an Apgar score? List the assessment parameters.

   _____

   _____

   _____

   _____

5. Define a cesarean delivery and list conditions that would indicate a reason for a cesarean delivery.

   _____

   _____

   _____

   _____

MATCHING I

Match each term with the correct definition.

1. _____ Herniation of the bladder into the vaginal wall.

2. _____ Mass that arises from the germ layers of the embryo that contains tissue remnants, including hair and teeth.

3. _____ Endometrial tissue growth outside of the uterine cavity.

4. _____ Fibrous, benign tumor of the uterus that usually arises from the myometrium.

5. _____ Excessive proliferation of tissue.

6. _____ Sexually transmitted disease or other disease arising from an infection that causes scarring of the fallopian tubes and adhesions in the abdominal and pelvic cavities.

7. _____ Bulging of intestinal tissue into a weakened posterior vaginal wall.

8. _____ Excessive menstrual bleeding.

9. _____ Persistent or bleeding ovarian follicle that fails to regress after ovulation.

10. _____ Diagnosed in women with persistent multiple cystic follicles.

11. _____ Weakness and stretching of the cardinal ligaments can result in this condition.

12. _____ Implantation of the embryo outside the intrauterine cavity.

a. Ovarian cyst

b. Hyperplasia

c. Polycystic ovary syndrome

d. Uterine prolapse

e. Cystocele

f. PID

g. Rectocele

h. Ectopic pregnancy

i. Dermoid cyst

j. Leiomyoma

k. Menorrhagia

l. Endometriosis

Match the surgical procedure with the correct definition.

1. _____ Removal of a circumferential core of tissue around the cervix.

2. _____ Ligation is performed to block the passage of ova through the tube and prevent implantation in the uterus.

3. _____ The removal of the uterus by a combined laparoscopic and vaginal approach.

4. _____ Surgical removal of the uterus and cervix through a transpelvic incision.

5. _____ Involves the dissection and wide removal of the uterus, fallopian tubes, ovaries, supporting ligaments, upper vagina, and pelvic lymph node chains.

6. _____ Complete removal of rectum, the distal sigmoid colon, the urinary bladder and distal ureters, and the internal iliac vessels and their lateral branches. All pelvic reproductive organs and lymph nodes, as well as the entire pelvic floor, pelvic peritoneum, levator muscle, and perineum, are removed.

7. _____ A fiber optic scope is inserted through the cervix and into the uterus.

8. _____ Removal of a benign leiomyoma of the myometrium to control bleeding and prevent pressure on other structures in the pelvis.

9. _____ Sharp and smooth curettes are used to remove the surface of the endometrium through a transvaginal approach.

10. _____ A transcervical approach is used to remove the uterus.

11. _____ Herniated tissue of the anterior and posterior vagina is reduced, and the vaginal walls are reconstructed.

12. _____ To create a functional vagina to facilitate sexual intercourse.

13. _____ A small, hollow tract that connects the bladder to the vagina.

14. _____ Shirodkar procedure performed on the cervical os to prevent spontaneous abortion of pregnancy.

15. _____ Wall may be everted and sutured to the skin to prevent recurrence.

16. _____ Surgical removal of the labia, as well as other structures of the vulva according to the extent of the pathology.

a. LAVH

b. TAH

c. Simple vulvectomy

d. Pelvic exenteration

e. Hysteroscopy

f. Cone biopsy of the cervix

g. Vesicovaginal fistula

h. Radical hysterectomy (Wertheim procedure)

i. Myomectomy

j. Bartholin gland cyst

k. Dilation and Curettage

l. Laparoscopic tubal ligation

m. Cerclage

n. Vaginal hysterectomy

o. Repair of a cystocele and rectocele

p. Vaginoplasty

MULTIPLE CHOICE

1. The first closing count of a cesarean section begins during closure of the:
   a. Uterus
   b. Peritoneum
   c. Fascia
   d. Subcutaneous

2. Which of the following is a hysterectomy clamp?
   a. Allen
   b. Heaney
   c. Harrington
   d. Pennington

3. Which of the following is a bladder retractor used during a cesarean section?
   a. DeLee
   b. O'Connor O'Sullivan
   c. Heaney
   d. Jackson

4. During a cesarean section, which of the following is a suction catheter used to suction the baby's mouth and nose?
   a. Asepto
   b. Yankauer
   c. Toomey
   d. DeLee

5. During a cesarean section, the incision in the uterus is extended with which of the following?
   a. Jorgensen scissors
   b. Heaney scissors
   c. Bandage scissors
   d. Jameson scissors

6. When a patient is positioned for a cesarean section, to prevent hypotension from pressure on the vena cava by the fetus, how is the patient positioned?
   a. Low lithotomy
   b. Modified left lateral with a wedge support under the patient's left hip
   c. Modified right lateral with a wedge support under the patient's right hip
   d. Supine

CASE STUDIES

1. *Many gynecology procedures are performed with the patient in the lithotomy position. What are the critical safety considerations for the lithotomy position?*

   1. _____

   2. _____

3. _____

4. _____

5. _____

6. _____

7. _____

8. _____

9. _____

10. _____

2. *You are scrubbed on a laparoscopic tubal ligation. Please answer the following.*

   a. Define laparoscopic tubal ligation.

   b. What position will the patient be in?

   c. What instrument trays will you use?

   d. What type of prep will be used?

e. How will you drape?

f. What type of setup will you use?

g. What anatomy do you need to be aware of?

24 Genitourinary Surgery

Student's Name _____

KEY TERMS

Write the definition for each term.

1. Arteriovenous fistula (or AV shunt): _____

2. Calculi: _____

3. Extracorporeal shockwave lithotripsy (ESWL): _____

4. Foley catheter: _____

5. Glomerular filtration rate (GFR): _____

6. Indwelling catheter: _____

7. Meatotomy: _____

8. Percutaneous: _____

9. Reflux: _____

10. Resectoscope: _____

11. Retrograde pyelography: _____

12. Specific gravity: _____

13. Staghorn stone: _____

14. Stent: _____

15. Tamponade: _____

16. Torsion: _____

17. Transurethral: _____

Identify the urinary catheters in the following figure, starting left to right.

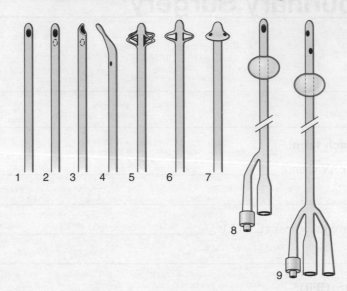

Modified from Walsh PC, Retik AB, Vaughan Ed, et al: *Campbell's urology*, ed 8, Philadelphia, 2002, WB Saunders.

1. _____

2. _____

3. _____

4. _____

5. _____

6. _____

7. _____

8. _____

9. _____

Identify the components of the male reproductive system.

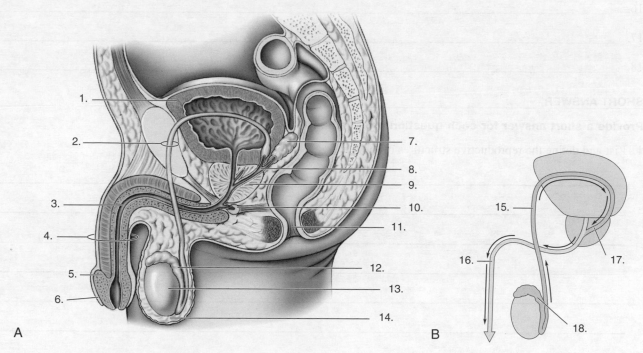

From Herlihy B, Maebius NK: *The human body in health and disease*, ed 2, Philadelphia, 2003, WB Saunders.

1. _____

2. _____

3. _____

4. _____

5. _____

6. _____

7. _____

8. _____

9. _____

10. _____

11. _____

12. _____

13. _____

14. _____

15. _____

16. _____

17. _____

18. _____

SHORT ANSWER

Provide a short answer for each question or statement.

1. List and define the reproductive structures of the male.

   _____

   _____

   _____

   _____

   _____

   _____

2. What is dialysis and how does it work?

   _____

   _____

   _____

   _____

   _____

   _____

Match each term with the correct definition.

1. _____ A small incision made in the urethra to reduce scarring or relieve a stricture.

2. _____ Fluid-filled cyst at the spermatic cord.

3. _____ Congenital defect in which the external urethral meatus is located on the bottom side of the penis.

4. _____ Fluid-filled sac arising in the layers of the tunica vaginalis of the testicle.

5. _____ Process by which urine is secreted from the bladder.

6. _____ A procedure in which ultrasonic sound waves are delivered from outside the body and used to pulverize kidney stones.

7. _____ Congenital condition in which the external urethral meatus is located on the top of the penis rather than the tip.

8. _____ Removal of all or part of the prepuce (foreskin) of the penis.

9. _____ Condition in which the foreskin cannot be retracted from the glans.

10. _____ Surgical creation of vascular access for patients undergoing hemodialysis.

a. Hypospadias

b. Hydrocele

c. Spermatocele

d. ESWL

e. Phimosis

f. Micturition

g. Epispadias

h. Urethrotomy

i. AV shunt

j. Circumcision

Match the term with the correct definition pertaining to the diagnostic test.

1. _____ Is performed to detect specific substances, both normal and abnormal, in urine.

2. _____ The presence or absence of specific substances in the blood reveals kidney function.

3. _____ Measures the rate of creatinine clearance from the blood.

4. _____ A test that assesses the elimination of urea from the liver.

5. _____ Tissue removed from the genitourinary (GU) tract for microscopic pathological testing.

6. _____ Is the preferred method for imaging tumors of the kidney.

7. _____ C-Arm real-time radiography.

8. _____ Radiographic studies using a contrast media to obtain radiographs of the renal pelvis and calyces.

9. _____ Radiograph of the kidney, ureters, and bladder used to outline structures of the urinary system.

10. _____ This study provides images of the bladder while it is emptying with use of contrast medium.

11. _____ Provides an extremely detailed assessment and is commonly used in the diagnosis of tumors.

12. _____ Radioisotope scanning in GU studies to detect metastasis arising from a primary tumor of the prostate.

13. _____ Retrograde injections are made using a catheter inserted into the ureter with contrast medium instilled in the catheter.

14. _____ One of the first-line imaging techniques used in GU medicine.

a. Tissue biopsy

b. Blood test

c. Computed tomography (CT)

d. Urinalysis

e. Blood urea nitrogen

f. Ultrasonography

g. Kidney, ureter, and bladder x-ray (KUB)

h. Glomular filtration rate (GFR)

i. Fluoroscopy

j. Magnetic resonance imaging (MRI)

k. IV urography

l. Micturating cystourethrogram (MCU)

m. Nuclear imaging

n. Retrograde ureteropyelogram

MULTIPLE CHOICE

1. Which procedure is removal of an enlarged prostate through an incision in the lower abdominal wall through the bladder?
   a. Transurethral resection of the prostate
   b. Open perineal prostatectomy
   c. Robot-assisted laparoscopic prostatectomy
   d. Suprapubic prostatectomy

2. The cortex of the kidney is covered with a strong fibrous tissue is called which of the following?
   a. Renal calyces
   b. Hilium
   c. Gerota's capsule
   d. Renal pyramids

3. Which of the following surgical procedures is removal of one or both testicles performed in cases of torsion or cancer?
   a. Phimosis
   b. Orchiectomy
   c. Hydrocelectomy
   d. Circumcision

4. Drainage and removal of a benign fluid-filled sac that develops in the anterior testis is which of the following?
   a. TURP
   b. Penectomy
   c. Orchiectomy
   d. Hydrocelectomy

5. Which of the following is a specimen evacuator collection device used to remove pieces of tumor during a TURP?
   a. Asepto
   b. Ellik
   c. Bulb
   d. Van Buren

6. Which of the following urethral catheters is used to traverse the urethra through an enlarged prostate?
   a. Coude
   b. Whistle tip
   c. Robinson
   d. Foley

CASE STUDIES

1. *You are about to scrub for a cystoscopy when the operating room supervisor delivers a surgical technology student to you and asks you to serve as her preceptor for the case. Your student has never seen a cystoscopy before, and you decide to describe the procedure to her before you start. What steps would you describe to her to explain the procedure?*

   a. _____

   b. _____

   c. _____

   d. _____

   e. _____

   f. _____

   g. _____

   h. _____

   i. _____

   j. _____

171

25 Ophthalmic Surgery

Student's Name _____

KEY TERMS

Write the definition for each term.

1. Accommodation: _____

2. Cataract: _____

3. Cryotherapy: _____

4. Diathermy: _____

5. Enucleation: _____

6. Evisceration: _____

7. Exenteration: _____

8. Focal point: _____

9. Glaucoma: _____

10. Keratoplasty: _____

11. Muscle recession: _____

12. Muscle resection: _____

13. Phacoemulsification: _____

14. Pterygium: _____

15. Refraction: _____

16. Spatula needle: _____

17. Strabismus: _____

SHORT ANSWER

Provide a short answer for each question or statement.

1. Explain the concept of refraction.

   _____

   _____

2. List and define the different types of diagnostic testing for the eye.

   a. _____

   _____

   _____

   b. _____

   _____

   _____

   c. _____

   _____

   _____

   d. _____

   _____

3. List the supplies needed for the sterile prep setup.

   a. _____

   b. _____

   c. _____

   d. _____

   e. _____

   f. _____

   g. _____

   h. _____

4. How should the instruments be cared for before, during, and after surgery?

_____

_____

_____

_____

5. What challenges does microsurgery present?

a. _____

_____

_____

b. _____

_____

_____

c. _____

_____

_____

6. List the guidelines for handling the microscope.

1. _____

2. _____

3. _____

4. _____

5. _____

6. _____

7. _____

8. _____

9. _____

10. _____

7. What is the protocol for the care of the microscope?

1. _____

2. _____

3. _____

8. What is the role of the surgical technologist during eye surgery?

a. _____

b. _____

c. _____

d. _____

e. _____

f. _____

g. _____

h. _____

i. _____

Match each term with the correct definition. You may use the same answer more than once or not at all.

1. _____ Performed for treatment of glaucoma to create a channel for the aqueous humor to drain from the anterior chamber.

2. _____ Procedure performed for detached retina.

3. _____ A process in which high-frequency sound waves are used to fragment tissue, such as a cataract.

4. _____ The procedure performed for a corneal transplant.

5. _____ Surgery in which the eye muscle is moved back to release the globe.

6. _____ Surgical shortening of an eye muscle to pull the globe into correct position.

7. _____ Creation of a permanent opening in the tear duct for drainage of tears.

8. _____ Surgical removal of the eyeball (globe) but eye muscles are left intact.

9. _____ Removal of nodal tissue arising from a sebaceous gland excised from the tarsal plate.

10. _____ Surgical removal of the contents of the eyeball, with the sclera and muscle attachments left intact.

11. _____ Removal of the entire contents of the eye socket, including the globe, muscles, fat, and eyelids.

12. _____ A technique in which a cold probe is used to freeze tissue, such as the sclera, ciliary body (for glaucoma), or retinal layers, after detachment.

13. _____ Low-power cautery used to mark the sclera over the area of retinal detachment.

a. Dacryocystorhinostomy

b. Trabeculectomy

c. Exenteration

d. Diathermy

e. Cryotherapy

f. Enucleation

g. Phacoemulsification

h. Muscle recession

i. Evisceration

j. Muscle resection

k. Chalazion

l. Scleral buckling

m. Keratoplasty

Match the drug with the brand name. You may use the same answer more than once or not at all.

1. _____ Constricts the pupil, used in intraocularly during anterior segment surgery.

2. _____ Stains the cornea yellow-green when used as a topical stain. When administered through an IV in angiography to diagnose retinal disorders

3. _____ Is a cholinergic, constricts the pupil, and is used topically to lower intraocular pressure in glaucoma.

4. _____ Injected subconjunctively for prophylaxis after eye procedures.

5. _____ Constricts the pupil.

6. _____ Mydriatic used to dilate the pupil but permit focusing for examination of the retina, testing refraction, and easier removal of the lens.

7. _____ Used to irrigate the eye to keep the cornea moist during surgery.

8. _____ Topical anesthetic applied directly to the eye providing loss of corneal sensation.

9. _____ Viscoadherent maintains a deep chamber for procedures of the anterior segment.

10. _____ Viscoelastic used to maintain separation between tissue and maintain pressure in the anterior chamber.

11. _____ Injectable anesthetic often used as a nerve block. Provides anesthesia of deep tissues.

12. _____ Osmotic diuretic administered intravenously to reduce intraocular pressure.

13. _____ Anticholinergic used for dilation of the pupil and for examination of the fundus and refraction.

14. _____ Adrenocorticosteroid anti-inflammatory agent injected subconjunctivally after surgery for prophylaxis.

a. Ancef, Kefzol

b. Occucoat

c. Miostat

d. Neo-Synephrine

e. Healon

f. Xylocaine

g. Tetracaine hydrochloride

h. BSS

i. Mydriacyl

j. Mannitol (osmitrol)

k. Decadron

l. Miotics

m. Pilocarpine hydrochloride

n. Fluorescein

MULTIPLE CHOICE

1. Ophthalmic sutures range in size from:
   a. 2-0 to 8-0
   b. 4-0 to 12-0
   c. 1-0 to 8-0
   d. 4-0 to 7-0

2. Which instrument is used to measure intraocular pressure?
   a. Sound
   b. Caliper
   c. Tonometer
   d. Depth gauge

3. Ophthalmic sponges are made from what type of material?
   a. Lint-free cellulose
   b. Oxidized cellulose
   c. Gelfoam
   d. Dry sponge sheets

4. During a lateral rectus resection, which suture is placed through the sclera as a traction suture?
   a. 7-0 nylon
   b. 3-0 nylon
   c. 6-0 vicryl
   d. 4-0 silk

5. An abnormal inversion of the lower eyelid, which causes the eyelashes to rub on the cornea.
   a. Strabismus
   b. Ectropion
   c. Entropion
   d. Chalazion

6. Which of the following is a circular cutting instrument that produces a tissue button during a corneal transplant?
   a. Spatula needle
   b. Vannas
   c. Westcott
   d. Trephine

7. Which of the following is a muscle hook?
   a. Jameson
   b. Vannas
   c. Westcott
   d. Trephine

8. An outwardly turned eyelid that creates an overflow of tears and exposes the conjunctiva, which becomes dry and irritated.
   a. Ectropion
   b. Enucleation
   c. Entropion
   d. Strabismus

CASE STUDIES

1. *You are a student assigned at a children's hospital and have been assigned to scrub in eye surgery with a preceptor who quizzes you frequently when you are ssigned to her. All of your cases in the room that day are to correct strabismus.*

    a. What is strabismus?

    b. What are the two common surgical procedures to correct strabismus? Provide a description of each procedure.

26 Surgery of the Ear, Nose, Pharynx, and Larynx

Student's Name _____

KEY TERMS

Write the definition for each term.

1. Cerumen: _____

2. Cholesteatoma: _____

3. Effusion: _____

4. Epistaxis: _____

5. Evert: _____

6. Hypertrophy: _____

7. Ossicles: _____

8. Ototoxic: _____

9. Packing: _____

10. Papilloma: _____

11. Paranasal sinus: _____

12. Paresis: _____

13. Perforation: _____

14. Phonation: _____

15. Polyp: _____

16. Sensorineural hearing loss: _____

17. Transcanal: _____

18. TM: _____

19. Transsphenoidal: _____

20. Tympanostomy tube: _____

SHORT ANSWER

Provide a short answer to each question or statement.

1. List methods of external examination of the ear and diagnostic procedures performed to evaluate the ear.

_____

_____

2. List functions and names of instruments used for nasal procedures.

a. Retractors

_____

_____

b. Knives

_____

_____

c. Elevators

_____

_____

d. Forceps

_____

_____

e. Rongeur

_____

_____

f. Gouge/chisel/osteotome

_____

_____

g. Rasp/saw

_____

_____

h. Scissors

_____

_____

181

3. List instruments needed for a tonsillectomy.

_____

_____

MATCHING I

Match each term with the correct definition.

1. _____ A benign tumor of the middle ear caused by shedding of keratin in chronic otitis media.

2. _____ Defect in the the tympanic membrane that can be caused by trauma or infection.

3. _____ Enlargement of the tonsils that can cause airway obstruction or sleep apnea.

4. _____ A benign epithelial tumor characterized by a branching or lobular shape.

5. _____ Fluid in the middle ear.

6. _____ Bleeding arising from the nasal cavity.

7. _____ Vibration of the vocal cords during speaking or vocalization.

8. _____ The most common cause of a break in the ossicle chain, which erodes the ossicles.

9. _____ Paralysis of a structure, such as vocal cord paresis.

10. _____ Excessive proliferation of mucosal epithelium.

11. _____ Hearing impairment arising from the cochlea, auditory nerve, or central nervous system.

12. _____ Can cause infection, otorrhea, bone destruction, hearing loss, and paralysis of the facial nerve.

a. Cholesteatoma

b. Papilloma

c. Polyp

d. Perforation

e. Epistaxis

f. Effusion

g. Hypertrophy

h. Paresis

i. Sensorineural hearing loss

j. Phonation

k. Cholesteatoma

MATCHING II

Match each term with the correct definition.

1. _____ A surgical opening is made in the tympanic membrane to release fluid.

2. _____ Close a small, nonhealing hole in the tympanic membrane.

3. _____ Surgical removal of a cholesteatoma and mastoid bone, with or without reconstruction.

4. _____ Removal of diseased bone, the mastoid air cells, and the soft tissue lining the air cell of the mastoid.

5. _____ The reconstruction of the ossicles to restore conduction to the oval window, performed to treat profound hearing loss related to sclerosis of the stapes.

6. _____ Is used to transmit external sound directly to the VIII cranial nerve, to treat sensineural hearing loss.

a. Mastoidectomy/ tympanomastoidectomy

b. Cochlear implant

c. Myringotomy

d. Tympanoplasty

e. Stapedectomy/ossicular reconstruction

f. Myringoplasty

MATCHING III

Match each term with the correct definition.

1. _____ Is performed to treat disease of the paranasal sinus, nasal cavity, and skull base and to improve nasal airflow.

2. _____ Maxillary sinus is exposed by making an incision in the gingival-buccal sulcus (the junction of the gum and upper lip).

3. _____ Removal of any bony obstruction at the frontal sinus to increase airflow through the nose.

4. _____ Surgical manipulation of the septum to return it to the correct anatomical position or to gain access to the sphenoid sinus for removal of a pituitary tumor.

5. _____ Is performed to reshape the external nose for aesthetic or functional purposes.

6. _____ Is performed to reduce ear, nose, and throat infection, and improve the airway.

7. _____ Surgical removal of the adenoids.

8. _____ Performed to reduce and tighten oropharyngeal tissue to improve obstructive sleep apnea.

9. _____ Endoscopic assessment of the larynx.

10. _____ Is performed in the emergency department, ICU, or operating room to create an airway for the patient.

a. Septoplasty

b. Endoscopic sinus surgery (ESS)

c. Tracheostomy/tracheostomy

d. Tonsillectomy

e. Caldwell-Luc

f. Laryngoscopy

g. Adenoidectomy

h. Turbinectomy/turbinate reduction

i. Rhinoplasty

j. UPP

MULTIPLE CHOICE

1. Which of the following is performed that involves removal of the larynx often including wide excision and tissue grafting as a part of the procedure?
   a. Total glossectomy
   b. Temporomandibular joint arthroplasty
   c. Radical neck dissection
   d. Laryngectomy

2. Procedure performed to treat malignant tumors; removal of all cervical lymph nodes and surrounding structures including the spinal accessory nerve, jugular vein, and sternocleidomastoid muscle.
   a. Radical neck dissection
   b. Laryngectomy
   c. Modified neck dissection
   d. Glossectomy

3. Which of the following is a type of salivary gland?
   a. Thyroid
   b. Parotid
   c. Cervical
   d. Adenexa

4. Which of the following is surgical removal of the entire tongue?
   a. Uvulopalatoplasty
   b. Tonsillectomy and adenoidectomy
   c. Modified radical neck dissection
   d. Glossectomy

5. Which of the following is an ear dressing consisting of several gauze sponges held in place with a molded plastic shield secured with Velcro straps?
   a. Colloid
   b. Fiberglass
   c. Glasscock
   d. Fluffs

CASE STUDIES

1. *If you are about to scrub for a radical neck dissection, you will have to know the extent of the dissection or the degree of pathology. What are the three types of neck dissection? What is involved in each?*

   a.

   b.

   c.

27 Oral and Maxillofacial Surgery

Student's Name _____

KEY TERMS

Write the definition for each term.

1. Arch bars: _____

2. Bicortical screw: _____

3. Blowout fracture: _____

4. Dentition: _____

5. LeFort I fracture: _____

6. LeFort II fracture: _____

7. LeFort III fracture: _____

8. Mastication: _____

9. Maxillomandibular fixation (MMF): _____

10. Occlusion: _____

11. Odontectomy: _____

12. Oromaxillofacial surgery: _____

13. Subciliary incision: _____

14. Transconjunctival incision: _____

LABELING

Facial trauma may involve the many bones of the face and frontal sinus. To increase your knowledge of the anatomy of the bones of the face, label the following diagram.

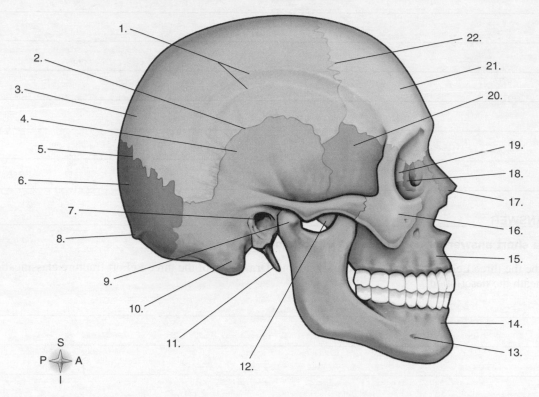

Modified from Thibodeau GA, Patt KT: *Anthony's textbook of anatomy and physiology*, ed 17, St Louis, 2003, Mosby.

1. _____

2. _____

3. _____

4. _____

5. _____

6. _____

7. _____

8. _____

9. _____

10. _____

11. _____

12. _____

13. _____

187

14. _____

15. _____

16. _____

17. _____

18. _____

19. _____

20. _____

21. _____

22. _____

SHORT ANSWER

Provide a short answer for each question or statement.

1. Describe the three LeFort facial fracture classifications. Draw each of the three LeFort fracture classifications underneath the description.

   1. _____

   _____

   _____

   2. _____

   _____

   _____

   3. _____

   _____

   _____

MATCHING

Match each term with the correct definition. You may use the same answer more than once or not at all.

1. _____ Procedure to wire the jaws in a closed position with arch bars.   a. Maxillomandibular fixation

2. _____ Chewing   b. ORIF

3. _____ Involved in "blowout" fractures.   c. Mastication

4. _____ Mandible   d. Upper jaw bone

5. _____ Maxilla   e. Orbital floor

6. _____ Open reduction and internal fixation of a fracture.   f. Frontal sinus

7. _____ Procedure performed to remove teeth.   g. Lower jaw bone

                                   h. Odontectomy

MULTIPLE CHOICE

1. Which of the following is a transverse fracture of the maxilla?
   a. LeFort I
   b. LeFort II
   c. LeFort III
   d. Odontectomy

2. Which gauge stainless steel wire is used for application of arch bars?
   a. 30–32 gauge
   b. 16–18 gauge
   c. 24–26 gauge
   d. 34–36 gauge

3. Which of the following is a pyramidal fracture of the maxilla?
   a. LeFort I
   b. LeFort II
   c. LeFort III
   d. Mandibular osteotomy

4. What must remain with the patient at all times postoperatively after arch bar application?
   a. Wire twisters
   b. Needle nose pliers
   c. Wire scissors
   d. Utility scissors

5. Which of the following fractures of the mid-face is the entire facial bone separated from the frontal bone through the zygoma?
   a. ORIF mandible
   b. ORIF maxilla
   c. LeFort I
   d. LeFort III

CASE STUDIES

1. *You are assigned to an ORIF repair of a mandible. Describe the purpose and steps of an open reduction and internal fixation of a mandibular fracture. What needs to be at the patient's bedside postoperatively?*

28 Plastic and Reconstructive Surgery

Student's Name _____

KEY TERMS

Write the definition for each term.

1. Aesthetic surgery: _____

2. Allograft: _____

3. Autograft: _____

4. Biological graft: _____

5. Biosynthetic graft: _____

6. Composite graft: _____

7. Debridement: _____

8. Dermatome: _____

9. Eschar: _____

10. Fasciotomy: _____

11. Full-thickness skin graft (FTSG): _____

12. Hypertrophic scar: _____

13. Keloid: _____

14. Mohs micrographic surgery: _____

15. Plication: _____

16. Porcine: _____

17. Ptosis: _____

18. Rule of nines: _____

19. Split-thickness (or partial-thickness) skin graft (STSG): _____

20. Synthetic grafts: _____

21. Undermine: _____

22. Xenograft: _____

LABELING

Label the following diagram. Name the type of skin graft in diagram A, then name the tissue layers. What type of skin graft is diagram B? Label the components of a hair follicle in diagram C.

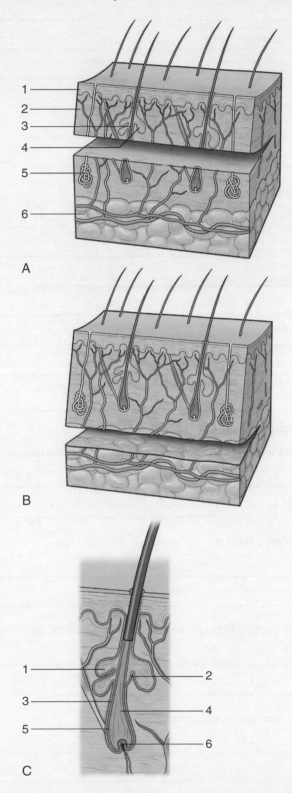

A. Type of skin graft: _____

    1. _____

    2. _____

    3. _____

    4. _____

    5. _____

    6. _____

B. Type of skin graft: _____

C. Label the structures of a hair follicle.

    1. _____

    2. _____

    3. _____

    4. _____

    5. _____

    6. _____

SHORT ANSWER

Provide a short answer to complete each question or statement.

1. What advances the aging process and what treatments are available to arrest the process?

_____

_____

2. What are the specific goals of plastic surgery?

_____

_____

3. Following an abdominoplasty or panniculectomy, what is the purpose of the postoperative position?

_____

_____

4. Describe the Rule of Nines and identify the percentages.

_____

_____

5. List types of dermatomes.

_____

_____

6. List the different types of skin graft materials.

_____

_____

7. List different types of implant materials or injectable fillers used for a mentoplasty.

_____

_____

8. Describe a debridement of a burn.

_____

_____

_____

MATCHING I

Match each term with the correct description.

1. _____ An unsevered graft raised from the donor site to provide coverage and vascularization to a soft tissue defect.

2. _____ A graft transferred from one individual (human) to another.

3. _____ A biological graft taken from one area of the body and transplanted to another area in the same patient.

4. _____ A biological graft consisting of more than one tissue type.

5. _____ A graft that contains only the dermis used to replace skin that has been lost as a result of trauma or disease.

6. _____ A graft derived from manufactured materials.

7. _____ A graft containing the dermis and epidermis used to cover a deep defect.

8. _____ Tissue taken from one species and grafted to another.

9. _____ Graft in which the entire graft is raised, excised, and transferred to another recipient site of the body.

10. _____ A graft derived from live tissue.

a. Allograft

b. Full-thickness skin graft

c. Biological graft

d. Xenograft

e. Split-thickness skin graft

f. Composite graft

g. Autograft

h. Synthetic graft

i. Pedicle graft

j. Free flap graft

MATCHING II

Match each term with the correct description.

1. _____ Is performed to remodel a previous scar or to remove a keloid.

2. _____ Is the removal of nonviable tissue from a burn or a nonhealing or traumatic wound.

3. _____ Reduction and removal of the loose apron of adipose tissue that arises from the lower abdomen.

4. _____ Resection of the eyelid to improve vision of the upper visual fields.

5. _____ Is performed to lift the supportive structures of the brow and alleviate drooping of skin, muscle, and fascia.

6. _____ Redundant and sagging supportive tissue of the face is reduced or modified to provide a more aesthetic appearance.

7. _____ Surgical modification of the external ear.

8. _____ Is performed to increase the size and improve the shape of the breast or create a new breast after mastectomy.

9. _____ Is performed to reduce excess breast tissue.

10. _____ Transverse rectus abdominis myocutaneous flap performed to reconstruct the breast without the use of implants.

11. _____ Is performed to remove excess deep fat with a cannula.

12. _____ Is performed to remove excess skin and adipose tissue from the abdominal wall.

13. _____ Performed to increase the height of the cheekbone for aesthetic purposes.

14. _____ Placement of a synthetic implant in the chin.

a. Malar augmentation

b. Liposuction

c. Abdominoplasty

d. Augmentation mammoplasty

e. Scar revision

f. Otoplasty

g. Panniculectomy

h. Brow lift

i. Debridement

j. TRAM

k. Blepharoplasty

l. Reduction mammoplasty

m. Rhytidectomy

n. Mentoplasty

MULTIPLE CHOICE

1. When performing a split-thickness skin graft, what is applied to the skin graft site to reduce friction?
   a. Vaseline
   b. Mineral oil
   c. Surgilube
   d. Lidocaine gel

2. During a split-thickness skin grafting procedure what is the graft mesher used for?
   a. Aerating the graft
   b. Increasing the surface area of the graft
   c. Improving contact between the graft and recipient site
   d. All of the above

3. Which of the following is treatment for a condition in which there is a pointed appearance of the ear at the top of the ear where it is normally rounded?
   a. Otoplasty
   b. Mentoplasty
   c. Correction of Stahl's ear
   d. Correction of syndactaly

4. Which is the technique of excising a malignant skin lesion by systematic removal of the margins and immediate microscopic examination, and additional tissue is removed until the margins of tissue are free of cancer cells?
   a. MOHS
   b. STSG
   c. FTSG
   d. DIEP

5. Which type of dressing is used after an STSG is placed to maintain contact between the skin graft and the tissue bed below it with a bolster that is secured over the graft with sutures?
   a. Glasscock
   b. Cast
   c. Stent
   d. Flat

CASE STUDIES

1. *Your patient is coming to surgery for debridement of a burn. Describe the different types of burns listed below using the American Burn Association classification system so you are familiar with the severity of the burn you will be treating.*

   a. Superficial partial-thickness, first-degree

   b. Partial-thickness, second-degree

   c. Full-thickness, second-degree

   d. Full-thickness, third-degree

29 Orthopedic Surgery

Student's Name _____

KEY TERMS

Write the definition for each term.

1. Alloy: _____

2. Aponeurosis: _____

3. Arthrodesis: _____

4. Bioactive implant: _____

5. Biocompatibility: _____

6. Biomechanics: _____

7. Broaches: _____

8. Cannulated: _____

9. Casting: _____

10. Closed reduction: _____

11. Comminuted: _____

12. Compartment syndrome: _____

13. Compression: _____

14. Cruciate: _____

15. Dislocation: _____

16. Distraction: _____

17. External fixation: _____

18. Internal fixation: _____

19. Open reduction: _____

20. Orthopedic system: _____

21. Press-fit: _____

22. Ream: _____

23. Reduction: _____

196

24. Replantation: _____

25. Tap: _____

26. Traction: _____

SHORT ANSWER

Provide a short answer for each question or statement.

1. What are the three stages of bone healing, and what occurs during each phase?

   a. _____

   b. _____

   c. _____

2. How are joints classified?

   a. _____

   b. _____

   c. _____

   d. _____

3. List the types of saws used in orthopedic surgery, including the movement/direction of the blade.

   _____

   _____

   _____

   _____

4. List the different types of instruments used in orthopedic surgery and give an example.

   _____

   _____

5. List the different types of fracture patterns and give an example of each.

   _____

   _____

   _____

   _____

6. Describe reduction and fixation of fractures.

   _____

   _____

7. List the parts of a screw and define.

_____

_____

8. List and define the different types of screws.

_____

_____

9. List the functions of a plating system.

_____

_____

10. List and define the different types of plates.

_____

_____

11. Define and give an example of the following: IM rod, wires and cables, K-wires, and Steinmann pins.

_____

_____

12. Traction is used for:

_____

_____

Describe two types of traction.

_____

_____

13. List and define the different types of arthroplasty materials used for joint replacement.

_____

_____

14. Describe the following drill attachments and accessories.

a. Burr: _____

_____

b. Chuck: _____

_____

c. Depth gauge: _____

_____

d. Drill bit: _____

_____

e. Drill guide: _____

_____

f. Reamer: _____

g. Shaver: _____

h. Tap: _____

_____

15. List hemostatic agents used on bone.

_____

_____

16. Describe laminar air flow.

_____

_____

17. List various dressing materials and uses applied in the operating room at the end of the case.

_____

_____

MATCHING I

Match each of the following types of joint.

1. _____ The fluid located in joints.

2. _____ Composed of a bony protuberance and an open collar component allowing rotation (first and second vertebrae of the neck).

3. _____ Has limited movement or a fixed articular surface such as between the bones of the cranium

4. _____ Has a rocker-and-cradle component, allowing extension and flexion only (elbow).

5. _____ The most freely movable type of joint allowing flexion, extension, abduction, adduction, rotation, and circumduction (hip).

6. _____ Freely movable synovial joint (shoulder).

7. _____ Joint in which the two components have a complimentary convex-concave shape in which the bones slide over each other. The body only has one, which is the thumb.

8. _____ Joint in which a small protrusion slides within a slightly elliptical component allowing flexion, extension, abduction, and adduction. (carpal bones of the wrist).

9. _____ Joint in which relatively flat surfaces of bone slide over each other (vertebrae).

10. _____ Joint in which bones are connected by cartilage and only slightly movable (symphasis pubis).

a. Hinge joint

b. Saddle joint

c. Gliding joint

d. Ball and socket joint

e. Pivot joint

f. Condyloid joint

g. Synovial

h. Diathrosis (synovial joint)

i. Amphiarthrosis (cartilaginous joint)

j. Synarthrosis (suture joint)

MATCHING II

Match the parts of the bone and different orthopedic pathology.

_____ 1. Compact bone found in the shaft of long bones, at the ends of joints, and in vertebrae where it is surrounds the softer cancellous bone.

_____ 2. Torn or detached tendon, ligament, or muscle often occurring as a sudden event or trauma.

_____ 3. Membrane covering the bones.

_____ 4. Partial or complete tearing away of tissue such as bone, tendon, muscle, or ligaments from the normal point of attachment.

_____ 5. Damage and disease of soft connective tissues caused by repetitive motion or repeated stress.

_____ 6. Found in the ends of long bone, containing red and yellow marrow, is also called spongy bone.

_____ 7. The ends of the long bones.

_____ 8. A break of the continuity of bone due to trauma or disease.

_____ 9. The middle shaft of the bone.

a. Avulsion

b. Fracture

c. Cortical bone

d. Cancellous bone

e. Periosteum

f. Diaphysis

g. Epiphysis

h. Overuse injury

i. Rupture

Match the procedure.

_____ 1. Performed to restore mobility to the hand and fingers by releasing constricted palmar fascia.

_____ 2. Fusion of the talocalcaneal, talonavicular, and calcaneocuboid joint.

_____ 3. Performed to treat a tear in the ACL to provide stability to the knee.

_____ 4. Reduction or removal of an enlarged hallux valgus.

_____ 5. Performed to reattach the labrum to the glenoid rim to correct recurrent glenohumeral dislocation.

a. Triple arthrodesis

b. Bankart procedure

c. Bunionectomy

d. Dupuytren contracture

e. Cruciate ligament repair

MULTIPLE CHOICE

1. Which is the longest bone in the body?
   a. Tibia
   b. Fibula
   c. Femur
   d. Phalanges

2. Application without an incision of an external fixator is which of the following?
   a. ORIF
   b. CREF
   c. CRIF
   d. OREF

3. Which of the following is a bone holding clamp?
   a. Cobb
   b. Langenbeck
   c. Hibbs
   d. Lowman

4. The single largest patient risk associated with casting is?
   a. Dupetryns
   b. Compartment syndrome
   c. Carpel tunnel
   d. Cardiac arrest

5. Which of the following is the most common site for bone graft harvesting?
   a. Ischium
   b. Femur
   c. Iliac crest
   d. Sacrum

CASE STUDIES

1. _Your patient has arrived for an arthroplasty. Describe patient risks associated with polymethylmethacrylate (PMMA), which is also called bone cement, and the technique used to reduce the hazards of PMMA._

2. *You have just been called in for orthopedic trauma. Knowing the types of bone fractures helps you choose the type of instrumentation needed for the repair. Working from left to right, label the fractures pictured in the following figure.*

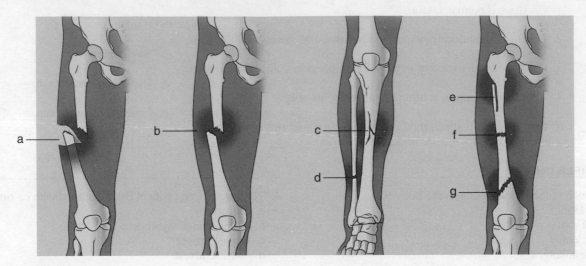

a. _____

b. _____

c. _____

d. _____

e. _____

f. _____

g. _____

30 Vascular and Microvascular Surgery

Student's Name _____

KEY TERMS

Write the definition for each term.

1. Aneurysm: _____

2. Angioplasty: _____

3. Arteriosclerosis: _____

4. Arteriotomy: _____

5. Atherosclerosis: _____

6. Bifurcation: _____

7. Doppler duplex ultrasonography: _____

8. Embolus: _____

9. Endarterectomy: _____

10. Endovascular: _____

11. Hemodialysis: _____

12. Hemodynamic: _____

13. Hybrid operating room: _____

14. In situ: _____

15. Infarction: _____

16. Intimal hyperplasia: _____

17. Intravascular ultrasound: _____

18. Ischemia: _____

19. Lumen: _____

20. Microsurgery: _____

21. Percutaneous: _____

22. Stent: _____

23. Thrombus: _____

24. Umbilical tape: _____

25. Venous stasis: _____

26. Vessel loop: _____

SHORT ANSWER

Provide a short answer for each question or statement.

1. List the structures of the blood vessel and define.

   _____

   _____

2. Define blood pressure and list factors that affect normal blood pressure.

   _____

   _____

3. List the major arteries of the body in their designated locations provided below.

   a. Thoracic cavity: _____

   b. Head: _____

   c. Upper extremeties: _____

   d. Abdomen: _____

   e. Lower limbs: _____

4. List the diagnostic procedures associated with peripheral vascular surgery.

   a. _____

   b. _____

   c. _____

   d. _____

5. List and give an example of instruments used in peripheral vascular surgery.

   a. _____

   b. _____

   c. _____

d. _____

e. _____

f. _____

6. List the sutures, accessories, vascular graft materials, and medications used for peripheral vascular surgery.

a. _____
_____

b. _____
_____

c. _____
_____

d. _____
_____

7. Define the following surgical procedures.

a. Endarterectomy
_____
_____

b. Intraoperative angiography
_____
_____

c. Angioplasty
_____
_____

d. Insertion of a vena cava filter
_____
_____

e. Vascular access for renal hemodialysis
_____
_____

205

f. Arteriovenous shunt

_____

_____

g. Arteriovenous fistula

_____

_____

h. Thrombectomy

_____

_____

i. Carotid endarterectomy

_____

_____

j. Abdominal aortic aneurysm

_____

_____

k. Aortobifemoral bypass

_____

_____

l. Axillofemoral bypass

_____

_____

m. Femorofemoral bypass

_____

_____

n. In situ saphenous femoropopliteal bypass

_____

_____

o. Femoropopliteal bypass

_____

_____

MATCHING I

Match the following.

1. _____ Carries blood back to the heart from the peripheral tissues.

2. _____ Carries oxygenated blood from the heart to the rest of the body.

3. _____ Moves blood to the lungs and back to the heart.

4. _____ Carries blood to all organs and tissues of the body except the lungs and then returns it to the heart.

5. _____ Carries deoxygenated blood from the heart to the lungs.

a. Arteries

b. Pulmonary arteries

c. Veins

d. Systemic circulation

e. Pulmonary circulation

MATCHING II

Match each disease process with the correct definition.

1. _____ Ballooning of an artery as a result of weakening of the arterial wall caused by atherosclerosis, infection, or anatomical defect.

2. _____ Clot of blood, air, or atherosclerotic plaque or fat that moves freely in the vascular system.

3. _____ Drop in blood pressure related to reduced blood or fluid volume.

4. _____ Abnormally high blood pressure.

5. _____ Blockage in an artery, leading to ischemia and tissue death.

6. _____ A stationary clot in the arterial or venous system.

7. _____ The most common form of arteriosclerosis, which causes plaque to form on the inner surface of an artery.

8. _____ Decrease or absence of blood supply to a localized area.

9. _____ Abnormal decrease in blood pressure.

10. _____ Disease characterized by thickening, hardening, and loss of elasticity of the artery walls.

a. Aneurysm

b. Arteriosclerosis

c. Atherosclerosis

d. Embolus

e. Hypotension

f. Hypovolemia

g. Hypertension

h. Infarction

i. Ischemia

j. Thrombus

MATCHING III

Match the following agents.

1. _____ Heparin

2. _____ Gelfoam

3. _____ Avitene

4. _____ Papaverine

5. _____ Surgicel

6. _____ Thrombin

a. Vasodilator

b. Topical hemostatic

c. Anticoagulant

MATCHING IV

Match the following; items may have more than one answer.

1. _____ Used to create a tubular space through tissue in which a graft can be threaded.

2. _____ Used for retraction of blood vessels.

3. _____ Glasses with mounted oculars used to magnify the surgical field.

4. _____ Used to prevent suture material from cutting through the arterial wall.

5. _____ Placed on tips of mosquito forceps to prevent damage to the suture on a double-ended suture.

a. Loupes

b. Shods/paws/boots

c. Loop

d. Umbilical tape

e. Pledget

f. Tunneler

MULTIPLE CHOICE

1. Which type of aneurysm is characterized by a hematoma that arises from a blood vessel?
   a. Fusiform
   b. Saccular
   c. Pseudo
   d. Dissecting

2. Which type of aneurysm is characterized by a bulging that is symmetrical?
   a. Fusiform
   b. Saccular
   c. Pseudo
   d. Dissecting

3. Which type of catheter is used to perform an embolectomy?
   a. Foley
   b. Filiform
   c. Coude
   d. Fogarty

4. Which type of aneurysm is characterized by its protrusion from one wall only?
   a. Fusiform
   b. Saccular
   c. Pseudo
   d. Dissecting

5. Which type of aneurysm results from a tear in the intima of the vessel that gives rise to splitting of the arterial wall?
   a. Fusiform
   b. Saccular
   c. Pseudo
   d. Dissecting

CASE STUDIES

1. *You are relieving the surgical technologist on a bilateral femoropopliteal bypass.*

   a. What is the first thing you should do when you scrub in?

b. What types of medication should you have on the field?

c. What types of sponges should you have on the field?

d. What extra sterile equipment should you have on the field?

e. What is the technique used in a femoropopliteal bypass?

f. After the case, what should you do?

31 Thoracic and Pulmonary Surgery

Student's Name _____

KEY TERMS _____

Write the definition for each term.

1. Apnea: _____

2. Arterial blood gases (ABGs): _____

3. Bleb: _____

4. Closed chest drainage: _____

5. Diffusion (oxygen): _____

6. Dyspnea: _____

7. Empyema: _____

8. Expiration: _____

9. Hemothorax: _____

10. Hypoxia: _____

11. Inspiration: _____

12. Perfusion (oxygen): _____

13. Pneumothorax: _____

14. Pulmonary function tests (PFTs): _____

15. Ventilation: _____

LABELING I

Draw a diagram of the bilateral lungs. Be sure to label your drawing. Include the following structures in your drawing.

Cartilaginous rings

Trachea

Apex

Primary bronchi

Superior lobe

Secondary bronchi

Tertiary bronchi

Bronchiole

Inferior lobe

Hilus

Base

Inferior lobe

Middle lobe

Superior lobe

SHORT ANSWER

Provide a short answer for each question or statement.

1. What organs and structures are located in the mediastinal space?

_____

_____

2. Explain the pleural cavity. Include in your explanation the pleural sac, pleural space, and negative pressure.

_____

_____

3. What diagnostic tests would be done on a patient who will undergo lung and respiratory surgical procedures?

_____

_____

_____

_____

_____

4. What position and incisions would most likely be used for patients undergoing pulmonary procedures?

_____

_____

5. List the equipment, supplies, and medication associated with thoracic and pulmonary surgery.

_____

_____

6. List the different types of instruments associated with thoracic and pulmonary surgery.

_____

_____

_____

7. Define the following surgical procedures associated with thoracic and pulmonary surgery.

a. Insertion of chest tube

_____

_____

_____

b. Rigid bronchoscopy

_____

_____

_____

c. Flexible bronchoscopy

_____

_____

_____

d. Mediastinoscopy

_____

_____

_____

e. VATS

_____

_____

_____

f. Endobronchial ultrasound

_____

_____

_____

g. VATS lung biopsy

_____

_____

_____

h. Lung volume reduction surgery

_____

_____

_____

i. Thoracotomy

_____

_____

_____

j. Lobectomy

_____

_____

_____

k. Pneumonectomy

_____

_____

_____

l. Decortication of the lung

_____

_____

_____

m. Lung transplantation

_____

_____

_____

MATCHING

Match the medical diagnosis with the correct surgical intervention. You may use the same answer more than once or not at all.

1. _____ Decortication of the lung

2. _____ Mediastinoscopy

3. _____ VATS

4. _____ Lung transplantation

5. _____ Lung volume reduction

6. _____ Lobectomy

7. _____ Chest tube insertion for bleeding

8. _____ Chest tube insertion for spontaneous collapse lung

9. _____ Thoracotomy

10. _____ Pneumonectomy

11. _____ Bronchoscopy

a. Dyspnea and hypoxia caused by pulmonary emphysema

b. Bronchitis

c. Removal of a small portion of lung tissue for pathological assessment with use of a thorascope

d. Thymus and lymph node biopsy to establish a diagnosis or determine cancer

e. End-stage pulmonary disease

f. Removal of a portion of the lung for treatment of cancer, cysts, localized infection, or trauma to a portion of the lung to prevent the spread of cancer

g. Hemothorax

h. Thoracic emergency such as an open or penetrating wound

i. Bronchiectasis, pulmonary obstruction, extensive or chronic abscess, or a palliative measure to slow the progression of cancer

j. Pneumothorax

k. Aspiration of a foreign body

l. Empyema

MULTIPLE CHOICE

1. Excessively deep respiration:
   a. Apnea
   b. Hyperventilation
   c. Hyperpnea
   d. Dyspnea

2. Cessation of breathing:
   a. Dyspnea
   b. Apnea
   c. Cyanosis
   d. Hypoventilation

3. Bluish tint to the skin seen in patients with poor oxygenation:
   a. Apnea
   b. Dyspnea
   c. Dysphasia
   d. Cyanosis

4. Difficulty or painful respiration:
   a. Dyspnea
   b. Dysphasia
   c. Diaphoresis
   d. Apnea

5. Which of the following is used during bronchoscopy
   to collect sputum of fluid samples?
   a. Ellik
   b. Toomey
   c. Lukens
   d. Chest drainage tube

CASE STUDIES

1. *Your patient has a lung disease and will have to undergo lung transplantation.*
   Answer the following questions about your patient and the procedure to better
   understand the operation.

   a. What disease processes might precipitate the patient's need for a transplant?

   b. In what position will your surgical patient be placed for the procedure?

   c. Will your patient need to go on bypass for the procedure?

32 Cardiac Surgery

Student's Name _____

KEY TERMS

Write the definition for each term.

1. Aneurysm: _____

2. Aortotomy: _____

3. Apex: _____

4. Arrhythmia: _____

5. Arteriosclerosis: _____

6. Atherosclerosis: _____

7. Bicaval cannulation: _____

8. Bradycardia: _____

9. Cardiac cycle: _____

10. Cardioplegia: _____

11. Coarctation: _____

12. Conduit: _____

13. Congenital: _____

14. Cross-clamp: _____

15. Diastole: _____

16. Endovascular repair: _____

17. Femoral cannula: _____

18. Fibrillation: _____

19. Infarction: _____

20. Ischemia: _____

21. Off-pump procedure: _____

22. Pacemaker: _____

23. Shunt: _____

216

24. Stenosis: _____

25. Sternotomy: _____

26. Systole: _____

27. Tachycardia: _____

28. Thoracoabdominal aortic aneurysm: _____

29. Thoracotomy: _____

30. Type A aortic dissection: _____

SHORT ANSWER

Provide a short answer for each question or statement.

1. What structures are in the thoracic cavity?

   _____

   _____

2. List the diagnostic tests associated with cardiac surgery.

   _____

   _____

3. List the equipment, supplies, and medication associated with cardiac surgery.

   _____

   _____

4. Describe the following items and equipment associated with cardiac surgery.

   a. Cardiac catheterization

   _____

   _____

   b. Vessel and patch grafts

   _____

   _____

   c. Prosthetic valves

   _____

   _____

217

d. Pacemaker

_____

_____

e. Cardiopulmonary bypass machine

_____

_____

5. Define the following surgical procedures.

a. Median sternotomy

_____

_____

b. CABG

_____

_____

c. Resection of a left ventricular aneurysm

_____

_____

d. Aortic valve replacement

_____

_____

e. Mitral valve repair and replacement

_____

_____

f. Resection of an aneurysm of the ascending aorta

_____

_____

g. Resection of an aneurysm of the ascending arch

_____

_____

h. Resection of an aneurysm of the descending thoracic aorta

_____

_____

i. Endovascular repair of a thoracic aneurysm

_____

_____

j. Insertion of an artificial cardiac pacemaker

_____

_____

k. Temporary pacemaker

_____

_____

l. Insertion and removal of an intraaortic balloon catheter

_____

_____

m. Left ventricular assist device

_____

_____

n. Heart transplantation

_____

_____

MATCHING

Match each term with the correct definition.

1. _____ Weakening of the heart muscle caused by obstruction of coronary arteries.

2. _____ Buildup of plaque or cholesterol deposits in the lining of the arteries.

3. _____ Chaotic disorganized stimulation of one or both atria that prevents atrial contraction.

4. _____ Disease of the arteries characterized by loss of elasticity and hardening of arterial walls.

5. _____ Weakening of the wall of an artery or the heart chamber, leading to thinning and ballooning.

6. _____ Cause for this would include valve disease, coronary artery disease, and congenital heart disease.

7. _____ Heart rate below 60 beats/min.

8. _____ Possible narrowing of aortic and mitral valve or valves.

9. _____ Cardiac muscle that beats abnormally fast.

a. Aneurysm

b. Arteriosclerosis

c. Atrial fibrillation

d. Bradycardia

e. Heart transplantation

f. Atherosclerosis

g. Myocardial infarction

h. Valve stenosis

i. Tachycardia

MULTIPLE CHOICE

1. Heart rate over 120 beats per minute:
   a. Atrial flutter
   b. Atrial fibrillation
   c. Ventricular fibrillation
   d. Ventricular tachycardia

2. Heart rate of 240 - 350 beats per minute:
   a. Ventricular tachycardia
   b. Atrial flutter
   c. Atrial fibrillation
   d. Ventricular fibrillation

3. Chaotic disorganized stimulation of one or both ventricles that does not pump the blood:
   a. Ventricular tachycardia
   b. Atrial fibrillation
   c. Ventricular fibrillation
   d. Bradycardia

4. Which of the following is a combination of congenital defects including pulmonary stenosis, ventricular septal defect, right ventricular hypertrophy, and displacement of the aorta?
   a. Tetralogy of Fallot
   b. Circle of Willis
   c. Wilm's
   d. Hirschsprung's

5. Which incision is used for incision for placement of a permanent pacemaker?
   a. Median sternotomy
   b. Thoracoabdominal
   c. Subxiphoid
   d. Subclavian

CASE STUDIES

1. *You are assigned to scrub for the surgeon who is performing grafting of the saphenous vein during a CABG. What supplies should you have available, and what are the steps of the procedure?*

33 Pediatric Surgery

Student's Name _____

KEY TERMS

Write the definition for each term.

1. Acquired abnormality: _____

2. Bolus: _____

3. Child life specialist: _____

4. Choana: _____

5. Coarctation: _____

6. Congenital: _____

7. Ductus arteriosus: _____

8. Embryonic life: _____

9. Exstrophy: _____

10. Fetus: _____

11. Genetic abnormality: _____

12. Homeostasis: _____

13. Isolette: _____

14. Magical thinking: _____

15. Mutagenic substance: _____

16. Nephroblastoma: _____

17. Neutral tube defect: _____

18. Omphalocele: _____

19. Pyloric stenosis: _____

20. Teratogen: _____

Provide a short answer for each question or statement.

1. Name three perioperative interventions used to maintain normothermia.

   a. _____

   b. _____

   c. _____

2. What is the surgical technologist's responsibility in reporting and calculating blood loss in pediatric patients?

   _____

   _____

3. Babies with esophageal atresia or a transesophageal fistula usually are low-birth-weight babies. Why?

   _____

   _____

4. What is Hirschsprung disease?

   _____

   _____

5. What is epispadias?

   _____

   _____

6. What is the primary differences regarding electrosurgery in the pediatric patient versus the adult patient?

   _____

   _____

7. List important considerations in pediatric anesthesia that differ physiologically and anatomically from adults.

   _____

   _____

   _____

   _____

8. List the specialty instrumentation related to pediatric surgery.

   _____

   _____

9. Thermoregulation is important during pediatric surgery. List and define the two risks that pediatric patients are particularly vulnerable to.

_____

_____

10. List the developmental stages of the child, and list a psychological characteristic.

_____

_____

_____

11. Define the following surgical procedures.
   a. Repair of a cleft lip

   _____

   _____

   b. Repair of a cleft palate

   _____

   _____

   c. Orchiopexy

   _____

   _____

   d. Pyloromyotomy

   _____

   _____

   e. Correction of choanal atresia

   _____

   _____

   f. Repair of pectus excavatum

   _____

   _____

   g. Nephrectomy in Wilms tumor

   _____

   _____

h. Repair of myelomeningocele

_____

_____

i. Correction of syndactyly

_____

_____

MATCHING

Match each medical diagnosis with the correct definition.

1. _____ Congenital blockage of an orafice or tubular structure.

2. _____ Chest wall deformity in which the sternum protrudes outward.

3. _____ Complex set of congenital anomalies involving the lower genitourinary tract and skeletal system.

4. _____ Congenital narrowing of the thoracic aorta that restricts blood flow to the lower body.

5. _____ Congenital anomaly in which abdominal viscera develops outside the body in which there is no membrane or peritoneal sac covering the contents.

6. _____ Wilms tumor.

7. _____ Congenital abnormality resulting from lack of folic acid in the mother's diet causing specific spinal cord defects such as spina bifida or anencephaly.

8. _____ Congenital anomaly in which the abdominal viscera develops outside the body contained within a peritoneal sac.

9. _____ A thickening of the pylorus that results in stricture at the gastric outlet.

10. _____ The opening of the urethra is fully exposed on the dorsum of the penis.

11. _____ Chemical change in the genetic structure that can cause skeletal deformity, microcephaly, and delayed development.

12. _____ Environmental agent (chemical or drug) that injures an embryo or a fetus.

a. Pyloric stenosis

b. Bladder exstrophy

c. Pectus carinatum

d. Atresia

e. Omphalocele

f. Neural tube defect

g. Coarctation of the aorta

h. Nephroblastoma

i. Gastroschisis

j. Epispadias

k. Teratogen

l. Mutagenic substance

CASE STUDIES

1. *There are items both in the environment and the diet of a pregnant woman that can cause developmental defects to the fetus. What are they, and what types of defects do they contribute to?*

34 Neurosurgery

Student's Name _____

KEY TERMS

Write the definition for each term.

1. Aneurysm: _____

2. Arteriovenous malformation (AVM): _____

3. Astrocytes: _____

4. Bone flap: _____

5. Craniectomy: _____

6. Cranioplasty: _____

7. Craniotomy: _____

8. Embolization: _____

9. Intracranial pressure (ICP): _____

10. Spondylosis: _____

11. Stereotactic: _____

SHORT ANSWER

Provide a short answer for each question or statement.

1. The brain is divided into three main sections. What are they?

   a. _____

   b. _____

   c. _____

2. Describe the three protective layers of membranes known as the meninges that protect the brain and spinal cord.

   a. _____

   b. _____

   c. _____

3. What are the lobes of the cerebrum, and what is each lobe responsible for controlling?

   a. _____

   b. _____

   c. _____

   d. _____

4. What are the major structures of the midbrain?

   _____

   _____

5. If it is necessary for a patient's hair to be removed for a cranial procedure, what is the protocol?

   _____

   _____

6. Why would your patient undergo a rhizotomy?

   _____

   _____

7. What is a disc herniation and why does it occur?

   _____

   _____

8. List the spinal vertebrae and how many vertebrae are in each section.

   _____

   _____

9. Hemostasis of the wound edge of an incision into the scalp for a craniotomy is achieved and maintained with the use of what?

   _____

   _____

10. What is CJD?

   _____

   _____

227

11. What are common diagnostic procedures that might be performed during the perioperative phase?

_____

_____

_____

_____

12. List the instruments associated with neurosurgery.

_____

_____

_____

_____

13. List two types of head stabilizers used for cranial surgery.

_____

_____

14. List two types of operating room tables used for neurosurgery.

_____

_____

15. Name a frame used for a posterior lumbar laminectomy.

_____

_____

16. Define the surgical procedure.

a. Craniectomy

_____

_____

b. Cerebral aneurysm

_____

_____

c. Arteriovenous malformation resection

_____

_____

d. Correction of craniosynostosis

_____

_____

e. Cranioplasty

_____

_____

f. Ventriculoperitoneal shunt

_____

_____

g. Transsphenoidal hypophysectomy

_____

_____

h. Stereotactic

_____

_____

i. Endoscopic ventriculoscopy

_____

_____

j. Anterior cervical discectomy with fusion – Open

_____

_____

k. Posterior cervical laminectomy

_____

_____

l. Lumbar laminectomy with discectomy

_____

_____

229

m. Microdiscectomy

_____

_____

n. Posterior lumbar interbody fusion

_____

_____

o. Rhizotomy

_____

_____

p. Ulnar nerve transposition

_____

_____

q. Carpal tunnel release

_____

_____

r. Thoracic corpectomy

_____

_____

MATCHING I

Match each term with the correct definition. You may use the same answer more than once or not at all.

1. _____ Narrow path that leads directly into the fourth ventricle.

2. _____ Outer tissue layer of the cerebrum.

3. _____ Continuous connection between the spinal cord and the pons.

4. _____ Layer of meninges that is closest to the brain.

5. _____ Ligament that connects one spinous process of a vertebra to another vertebra.

6. _____ Small bulges that occur throughout the surface of the cerebrum.

7. _____ Large, deep furrows in the cerebrum.

8. _____ Covers and protects the brain.

9. _____ Area of brainstem responsible for vital functions of the circulatory system, respiration, and heart rate.

10. _____ The outermost layer of the meninges.

a. Skull

b. Cerebral aqueduct

c. Medulla oblongata

d. Cerebral cortex

e. Medulla

f. Gyri

g. Fissures

h. Ligamentum flavum

i. Pia mater

j. Dura mater

MATCHING II

Match the following cranial nerves.

1. _____ Controls lateral movement of the eye.

2. _____ Controls muscles of the tongue.

3. _____ Has two parts: a cranial portion and a spinal portion.

4. _____ Sense of smell.

5. _____ Sensations of the face, forehead, mouth, nose, and top of the head.

6. _____ Sense of taste and pharyngeal movement.

7. _____ Conveys impulses for sight.

8. _____ Controls hearing and equilibrium.

9. _____ Controls muscles that move the eye and iris.

10. _____ Controls muscles of the face and scalp, tears, and salivation.

11. _____ Innovates pharyngeal and laryngeal muscles, heart, pancreas, lungs, and digestive systems.

12. _____ Controls oblique muscles of the eye.

a. I (Olfactory)

b. II (Optic)

c. III (Oculomotor)

d. IV (Trochlear)

e. V (Trigeminal)

f. VI (Abducens)

g. VII (Facial)

h. VIII (Vestibulocochlear)

i. IX (Glossopharyngeal)

j. X (Vagus)

k. XI (Accessory)

l. XII (Hypoglossal)

MULTIPLE CHOICE

1. Which of the following is a cerebral aneurysm clip?
   a. Filshie
   b. Falope
   c. Yasargil
   d. Hulka

2. Which of the following are small square felted sponges used to control bleeding on neural and vascular tissue?
   a. Tonsil
   b. Cottonoid
   c. Peanut
   d. Pusher

3. Which of the following is a spinal retractor?
   a. Taylor
   b. Charnley
   c. Lowman
   d. Lewin

4. When closing for a craniotomy, which is the first layer that is closed?
   a. Galea
   b. Skin
   c. Subcutaneous
   d. Dura

CASE STUDIES

1. *Your patient's illness has been recently diagnosed as an endocrine-dependent malignant tumor of the pituitary gland.*

   a. What signs or symptoms did your patient most likely have when she arrived at the physician's office?

   b. What procedure will the surgeon suggest to the patient as a potential cure?

   c. How will the surgeon describe to the patient the potential postoperative complications for this procedure?

   d. Where will the incision be?

e. Once the tumor is resected, what will be used to pack the floor of the sella to prevent or manage a CSF leak?

2. *Your surgical case today is an open craniotomy for removal of a tumor. The surgeon is going to create and remove a bone flap for access to the tumor. As the scrub, what is your responsibility with regard to the bone if it is removed from the patient?*

35 Emergency Trauma Surgery

Student's Name _____

Write the definition for each term.

1. Advance Trauma Life Support (ATLS): _____

2. Algorithms: _____

3. Autotransfusion: _____

4. Blunt injury: _____

5. Cardiac rupture: _____

6. Cardiac tamponade: _____

7. Coagulopathy: _____

8. Compartment syndrome: _____

9. Contusions: _____

10. Damage control surgery: _____

11. Definitive diagnosis: _____

12. Definitive procedure: _____

13. Exsanguinating: _____

14. Flail chest: _____

15. Focused assessment with ultrasound for trauma (FAST): _____

16. Hemorrhagic shock: _____

17. Hemothorax: _____

18. Metabolic acidosis: _____

19. Occult injury: _____

20. Penetrating injury: _____

21. Pneumothorax: _____

22. Resuscitation: _____

234

SHORT ANSWER

Provide a short answer for each question or statement.

1. Describe damage control surgery and the goals of damage control surgery.

   _____

   _____

2. List the trauma system and define.

   _____

   _____

   _____

3. List and define the lethal triad.

   _____

   _____

4. List the ATLS principles of trauma management.

   _____

   _____

5. List and define the A, B, C, D, E primary patient assessment performed by first responders.

   _____

   _____

6. List and give an example of the preoperative care of the patient.

   _____

   _____

7. List the proper way to manage the sterile field in an emergency trauma.

   _____

   _____

8. Describe disseminated intravascular coagulation (DIC).

   _____

   _____

   _____

9. How should forensic evidence be handled?

   _____

   _____

   _____

10. List and give an example of the following surgical procedures related to trauma.

a. Laparotomy with staged closure

_____

_____

b. List steps of damage control techniques for abdominal trauma.

_____

_____

c. Abdominal compartment syndrome

_____

_____

d. Orthopedic trauma

_____

_____

e. Emergency treatment of orthopedic fractures

_____

_____

f. Thoracic injury

_____

_____

g. Blunt cardiac rupture

_____

_____

h. Penetrating cardiac wound

_____

_____

i. Flail chest

_____

_____

j. Aortic injury

_____

_____

k. Hemothorax

_____

_____

l. Laceration of the lung

_____

_____

m. Trauma of the brain and spinal cord

_____

_____

n. Trauma related to major peripheral vascular trauma

_____

_____

MULTIPLE CHOICE

1. Prehospital care of the trauma patient morbidity and mortality are partially related to the time elapsed between the first critical hour of care after injury is referred to as the:
   a. ABCDE
   b. Resuscitation
   c. Secondary survey
   d. Golden hour

2. Which of the following is a hematoma between the dura and the brain?
   a. Intracerebral hematoma
   b. Subdural hematoma
   c. Subarachnoid hematoma
   d. Arteriovenous hematoma

3. Which of the following is the most common cause of penetrating brain injury?
   a. Knife wounds
   b. Motor vehicle accident
   c. Gunshot wounds
   d. Traumatic subarachnoid hemorrhage

4. Which of the following would most likely cause thoracic injuries, sternal and rib fractures, flail chest, cardiac contusion, aortic injuries, and hemo- or pneumothorax during a motor vehicle accident?
   a. Windshield
   b. Ejection from the vehicle
   c. Rollover
   d. Steering wheel

5. Which of the following is vascular failure caused by severe blood loss and the most common cause of mortality in trauma?
   a. Hemorrhagic shock
   b. Hypothermia
   c. Metabolic acidosis
   d. Hypokalemia

Complete the following chart.

Techniques for Temporary Abdominal Closure

Technique	Description	Mechanism
1. _____	A perforated plastic sheet covers the viscera, and a sponge is placed between the fascial edges. The wound is covered by an airtight seal, which is pierced by a suction drain connected to a suction pump and fluid collection system.	The (active and adjustable) negative pressure supplied by the pump keeps constant tension on the fascial edges while it collects excess abdominal fluid and helps resolve edema.
2. _____	A perforated plastic sheet covers the viscera, damp surgical towels are placed in the wound, and a surgical drain is placed on the towels. An airtight seal covers the wound, and negative pressure is applied through the drain.	The negative pressure keeps constant tension on the fascial edges, and excess fluid is collected.
3. _____	Two opposite Velcro sheets (hooks and loops, one on each side) are sutured to the fascial edges. The Velcro sheets connect in the middle.	This technique allows for easy access and stepwise reapproximation of the fascial edges.
4. _____	The viscera are covered with a sheet (e.g., ISODrape, Microtek [Microban], Huntersville, NC). Horizontal sutures are placed through a large-diameter catheter and through the entire abdominal wall on both sides.	The sutures keep tension on the fascia and may be tightened to allow staged reapproximation of the fascial edges. This may be combined with a vacuum system.
5. _____	A sterile x-ray film cassette bag or sterile 3-L urology irrigation bag is sutured between the fascial edges or the skin and opened in the middle.	This is an easy technique that allows for easy access. The bag may be reduced in size to approximate the fascial edges.
6. _____	An absorbable or nonabsorbable mesh or sheet is sutured between the fascial edges. Examples are Dexon, Marlex, or Vicryl mesh. Examples of sheets are Silastic or silicone sheets.	The mesh or sheet may be reduced in size to allow for reapproximation. Nonresorbable meshes may be removed or left in place at the end of the open abdominal period.

Modified from Diaz J, Duton W, Miller R: The difficult abdominal wall. In Townsend CM Jr, Beauchamp RD, Evers BM, Matto x KL, editors: *Sabiston textbook of surgery*, ed 19, Philadelphia, 2012, WB Saunders.

36 Disaster Preparedness and Response

Student's Name _____

KEY TERMS

Write the definition for each term.

1. Agency for Healthcare Research and Quality (AHRQ): _____

2. All-hazards approach: _____

3. American Red Cross: _____

4. Bioterrorism: _____

5. Declared state of emergency: _____

6. Disaster: _____

7. Disaster recovery: _____

8. Emergency: _____

9. Federal Emergency Management Agency (FEMA): _____

10. Logistics supply chain: _____

11. Mass casualty event: _____

12. Mitigation: _____

13. National Fire Protection Agency (NFPA): _____

14. Natural disaster: _____

15. Pandemic: _____

16. Shelter-in-place: _____

17. Surge capacity: _____

18. Vulnerability: _____

SHORT ANSWER

Provide a short answer for each question or statement.

1. What is the difference between a disaster and an emergency?

   _____

   _____

2. List types of natural disasters.

   _____

   _____

3. List types of intentional violence/terrorism disasters.

   _____

   _____

4. What is bioterrorism?

   _____

   _____

5. Define the three levels of disasters.

   _____

   _____

6. What role does the community play in disaster preparation?

   _____

   _____

7. List the primary objectives of a local disaster plan.

   _____

   _____

MATCHING

Match each term with the correct definition.

_____ 1. An important activity in infection control during a disaster.

_____ 2. Ensures that a disaster response is consistent with the doctrines and laws of the country.

_____ 3. Way of moving people away from a disaster to protect them from catastrophic morbidity and mortality.

_____ 4. A process of putting family members in contact with each other during or after a disaster.

_____ 5. Social and psychological assistance needed in every disaster.

_____ 6. Protects people from extreme weather, including environmental conditions.

_____ 7. Form the process of transport and distribution of materials, goods, food, and other necessary supplies.

_____ 8. A designated area for placing the dead, far from the emergency department outside the building to avoid patients and the public.

a. Shelter

b. Evacuation

c. Temporary morgue

d. Logistics

e. Mental health needs

f. Health messages in the community

g. Department of Homeland Security

h. Reunification

MULTIPLE CHOICE

Choose the most correct answer for each question or statement.

1. _____ is a process in which casualties are given emergency medical treatment according to the probability of their survival.
   a. Surge capacity
   b. Communication
   c. Triage
   d. Medical facility evacuation

2. A major health facility has the ability to _____ using satellite or high frequency radio.
   a. Analyze surge capacity
   b. Communicate
   c. Perform triage
   d. Evacuate injured people

3. _____ of a medical facility may sometimes be necessary because of structural hazards or immediate threat from fire, chemical, or bioterrorism.
   a. Surge capacity
   b. Communication
   c. Triage
   d. Evacuation

4. _____ is the ability of a health care facility to quickly increase its capability to receive and treat patients.
   a. Surge capacity
   b. Communication
   c. Triage
   d. Medical facility evacuation

5. Roles are assigned using a *job action sheet* (JAS). This is a tool used to define:
   a. Surge capacity
   b. Staff assignments
   c. Triage
   d. Medical facility management team

6. During a disaster, individual health care workers may be asked to:
   a. Perform tasks outside their scope of practice
   b. Perform tasks outside their usual role
   c. Perform management tasks even though they have no experience
   d. Be a spokesperson for the hospital

7. During a disaster, the press and other media require:
   a. Food and water from the health facility
   b. The ability to examine patients
   c. Lists of the dead
   d. A designated media representative to work in the communication area to control accuracy in reporting

CASE STUDIES

1. *Read the following case study and answer the question based on your knowledge of the health care disaster plan.*

A mass casuality event has occurred in the community. The hospital has activated its emergency plan, including the deployment of all staff, and you have been informed to report to the hospital.

What would you imagine your role as a surgical technologist to be during a mass casuality event?

NOTES

NOTES

NOTES

NOTES